Life Simplified

A weekly guide to creating a life you love!

Leslie Gail

authorHOUSE®

AuthorHouse™
1663 Liberty Drive, Suite 200
Bloomington, IN 47403
www.authorhouse.com
Phone: 1-800-839-8640

First published by AuthorHouse   12/22/2008

ISBN: 978-1-4389-3850-9 (sc)

Printed in the United States of America
Bloomington, Indiana

This book is printed on acid-free paper.

*This book is dedicated to my mother, Susan,
who was truly an angel on earth.*

Contents

Acknowledgments

I am grateful to have so many blessings in my life, including many people to thank and acknowledge. Without the love and support of my family and friends, this book would not have been created.

I need to begin by thanking the love of my life, Roger. Without your love and unconditional support, I would not be the woman I am today. Thank you, especially, for the countless number of hours you occupied our children, so that I could devote the time and energy needed to bring this book to life.

I am very fortunate to have a father who gave me the foundation to live a rich and prosperous life. Your passion for life is such an inspiration to everyone you meet. Thank you for igniting a desire to always reach for the stars.

Without my family I would not have created this sacred life. To my sister Tami: what can I possibly say to the woman I admire and respect more than anyone? You are a constant source of support and pure joy. Just being around you brings a peace I cannot explain. To my brother Mark, who has always been one of my biggest cheerleaders: Mark, thank you for your honesty and unconditional love. And to my brother-in-law Brett and sister-in-law Rachel Ann, I could never have dreamed of gaining another sister and brother whom I love and respect as much as you two.

I would love to also dedicate this book to my two angels on earth, my children Cameron and Morganne. Raising the both of you has been the biggest blessing and honor of my life. I have learned so much about myself just from experiencing life through your eyes. I am constantly inspired to write and talk about things that directly relate to you two. You are both pure joy and light and I thank you for giving me the time and space to write this book.

To all of my friends, thank you for being part of my life! Growing up, I strived to have a handful of good friends like my mother had. I can honestly say that I am so grateful to all the women that I call friends. You have supported me and nurtured me through this process, and all a while accepted me as-is. Thank you for coming into my life and bringing wonderful memories and cherished experiences along the way. A special thanks to my dear friends Katherine and Jill for offering honest feedback while creating this book.

Finally, I need to thank my clients for teaching me every step of the way. Every single client I have been blessed to work with has taught me about life and meaning. You may think that I was the teacher in our relationship, but you have each brought something unique and special to my life. Thank you!

About the Author

I realized a long time ago that I viewed life a little differently than most people. I was, and still am, extremely sensitive and tuned in to the happenings of the world. I wear my heart on my sleeve and feel others' emotions and pain. I never understood why people got so upset over fairly trivial matters. I have never understood why people make a mountain out of a molehill. I guess I tend to look at the larger picture at hand and have an easy way of putting things into perspective. This, of course, always attracted friends to come to me for advice and insight. This was the beginning of my path in life.

Growing up with a psychiatrist for a father and a loving stay-at-home mom, we were given the gift of expression and freedom to explore the world. As my mother battled illnesses on and off from the time I was a very little girl, I learned a great deal about life and death. She taught me more in the 24 years I had her in my life than most people learn in a lifetime. In the years that I was blessed to have her in my life, I learned the following: power of friends, perseverance, positive attitude, being in the moment, giving it your all, never giving up, living life to the fullest, and most importantly, being true to yourself and your passions. She ultimately taught by example how to live a life you were meant to live.

I never take for granted all of the blessings I have in my life, for you never know what tomorrow will bring. This journey with my mother led me to follow my instinct and intuition. It taught me to follow that feeling that we are all born with, for it will never guide you in the wrong direction. It is a matter of fine tuning and really listening, not ignoring, the signals that are always there for your benefit. This ultimately led me to Life Coaching.

I first heard about coaching from my sister, who was a coach in Los Angeles. At some point I thought it sounded intriguing. What interested me about coaching was the proactive approach to working with clients. Instead of clients coming in every week discussing what was not working in their lives, and then not doing much about it, I, as their coach would be able to help them move forward. They could apply tools and simple techniques to move them past their comfort zones, thus propelling them forward in their life.

I received my certification as a life coach soon thereafter, and then moved at a fairly quick pace with my business. I believe we are all meant to do something special with our lives, and this I believe was what I was meant to do. Looking back at my life up until that point, everything was a stepping stone to get me to where I am. I began fine tuning my skill, and doors started opening. Opportunities presented themselves to me and I was in the full swing of a thriving and fulfilling practice. Let me be clear however, that things didn't just happen on their own accord. I created everything by asking for what I wanted and being extremely persistent.

Let me give you some examples. I write weekly articles entitled "Monday Morning Tips," that I send via e-mail to my client and subscriber base. You can sign up directly at www.newlifefocus.com . I contacted the newspaper in Denver, Colorado and inquired about having these articles published. Before I knew it, they were publishing them on a regular basis. I then contacted the producer at a major morning radio show and was invited to appear on their show. I clicked very quickly with the DJ's and became a regular expert guest. Things were happening at a nice pace and it was time to make new progress. I contacted a producer at the NBC affiliate, which resulted in a short segment that was aired on the newscast. Months after that, I began a weekly segment on the ABC affiliate, offering their viewers simple yet practical tips on improving their lives.

All of these things are examples that your life is what you make of it. I took advantage of my outgoing personality and ability as a coach to connect with people on a larger basis. My journey up to this point has been extremely enlightening and I am blessed with an amazing family and group of friends. My life experiences all go into the advice I give my clients, and my passion for living a purposeful life radiates to all those I come across. I currently reside in Denver, Colorado with my husband and two children.

Introduction

The fact that you picked up this book tells me so much about you as a person. You are feeling a variety of things in your life, and you are looking for a little support and guidance. I commend you for taking control of your life; for being open to making changes. It is easier to blame others for your circumstances, so it truly says something about the type of person you are for taking responsibility for your life. We all hit periods in our lives when we are bombarded with transition or unexpected situations. The true survivors are the ones who acknowledge what is happening, learn from the situation, and move on.

This book is an accumulation of tips to propel you forward in your life at an uncomplicated speed. Many people have areas of their life where they are unsatisfied. You may be unhappy with your career, or you may feel unbalanced. You may be seeking a fulfilling relationship or need some help creating boundaries in your life. Whatever the situation, this book will give you the support and structure to make these necessary changes.

The chapters range from getting rid of emotional and physical clutter in your life, to embracing gratitude in your life, to living a life of no regrets. There is a wide variety of topics that ultimately will improve the quality of your life. Each chapter gives a basic overview of the topic and then includes three action steps. When you apply the action steps, they will propel you forward in your life. I am a firm believer that action is ultimately what creates change in your life. You can talk the talk, but until you are willing to apply the tools and act upon them, you will remain stuck. I have also included stories from clients past and present. All of the names have been changed to respect their privacy.

There is a basic order to the book that helps you clean up certain areas of your life first prior to embarking on major life changes. I am a firm believer that you need to fix the problem instead of just placing a band-aid on the wound. You can fix problems by creating solid foundations, and you can accomplish this by de-cluttering and simplifying your life, creating boundaries, asking for your needs to be met, and plugging passion back into your routine. This is all vital if you want to move forward healthy and strong-minded. When you are at a healthy place you are able to attract all that you desire into your life. Instead of chasing what you want, you attract it *to* you.

How many of you are tired of trying so hard to create the life you envision for yourself? How nice would it be if you attracted everything to you by putting those intentions to motion? I believe that is possible with a genuine desire, commitment, and consistency to the process. Follow the advice in this book and you will notice a shift in your awareness. This will then lead to opportunities, happiness, and a sense of joy again in your life.

This book breaks down the topics into a weekly focus. Most individuals do better on short term projects than looking at the larger picture at hand. By focusing every week on one topic, this allows you to move forward one week at a time. You can look at the Table of Contents and follow A to Z, in that order. If you make one change every week in your life, within six months you will have a dramatically improved life and way of thinking. Just take it one week at a time. I have also included a section called ***Simplified Help.*** In this portion of each chapter, I will address certain concerns some of you may have regarding the topic at hand. If you are struggling with taking the needed action, this area will address some of those apprehensions. I also include in every chapter ***Simplified Affirmations***. You can read these affirmations aloud or create your own. Every chapter has its own set of affirmations that are geared toward putting your action into intention form.

Go out and buy a journal that you can use to document some of the exercises in this book. You will want one place where you can keep all of your writings, all of your thoughts, so that you can look back at any time and remember why you documented certain things. This will be your self discovery bible of sorts, so treat it with kindness and thought. I will be by your side throughout this journey and I am humbled that you have chosen this book to guide you to the next chapter in your life.

I hope this book gives you the support and tools to make positive life changes. All I ask of you is to give yourself the opportunity to succeed. Use this book to create action in your life. The purpose of this book is not only to read the book and put it away. It is an interactive book to apply simple tools in your life, thus creating forward momentum. Trust that you picked up this book for a reason and be open to the changes awaiting you!

Week 1

Always De-clutter Life First

How often do you walk into your home, office, or bedroom and instantly feel tension build up in your body? Imagine clutter everywhere, piles here and piles there. You feel lost as to how to begin organizing everything. You see these tasks as overwhelming and daunting, so you don't even begin, right? The disorganization we see around us is often related to the internal chaos in our lives. When your responsibilities and obligations have exceeded a healthy level, it permeates into your physical environment. Imagine entering your home or office with everything in its place. Would the tension dissipate? It is a tangible possibility to create this environment by breaking down the larger tasks into smaller and more manageable ones.

A former client, Laura, was drowning in the clutter and chaos of her life. As a mother of three, she was constantly in transit from one place to another, and in the process her home was being neglected. Amidst her clutter, she was unable to focus on the things she valued, like her family, losing sight of them while in survival mode. She realized something needed to change, and that is when she came to me for help and guidance. I told her that before embarking on the larger goals at hand, we needed to first clean up her life from the inside out. We needed to get rid of the clutter, both physically as well as emotionally, before moving forward.

Laura listed everything that needed to get controlled in her home, whether basic or elaborate. The list ranged from getting rid of old clothes to organizing recipes in her kitchen. While it may seem simplistic, collectively these things were all holding her back from fully enjoying life. By starting with little things she was able to eliminate unnecessary clutter and realign her focus from what she wasn't getting done to what she was most proud of - her family and herself.

Creating an environment that is conducive to success means going back to the basics. This is an important first step when embarking on life changes. Create a fresh environment first, and then you will be able to embark on the larger issues in your life with a clear mind.

Tips for the Week

1. Make a list

Create a master list of all the different areas that you need to address. The more specific, the better. Remember, you will be tackling one area at a time. Do not get overwhelmed by everything you have to do. This list will enable you to break down the different focus areas into more manageable goals. Feel free to divide your list into subcategories. Some areas to address might be your kitchen counters, master bedroom closet, home office space, or organizing your garage.

2. Pick and choose

Now that you have your master list, break it down by priority. If something has been weighing on you, mark that as a top priority. You need to focus on one area first, conquer it, and then move on. Do not try a little here and a little there. Do not move on to another project until the one at hand is complete. Feel free to mark your list from A to Z with A taking top priority. Sometimes we want to do everything at the very moment that we think of it. Then what happens? Nothing gets accomplished because you are scattered and moving from project to project without ever completing anything. Accept the fact that you will accomplish so much more when you commit to one area at a time. The feeling of accomplishment will motivate you to keep going.

3. Structure it

You need to set aside time on a regular basis to make continual progress. Just like you would set aside time to get ready in the morning, you need to set aside designated time to work on the project at hand.

Choose a time that works well with your schedule and get to work. Maybe set 30 minutes a day of uninterrupted time to focus and make progress. Set a timer if that helps. Once the timer goes off, you have the choice to continue working or walk away and continue later. The majority of people who set a timer will keep working even after it goes off. You may be in a positive groove, so why stop? Do what feels right to you.

Whenever I feel the clutter start to pile up in my home or office, it's crucial that I set aside time to get it back to order. I am so much more productive in all elements of my life when things look and feel clean. It is a small amount of time to devote in terms of feeling better physically and emotionally. There are many times when I think I will only devote a small amount of time to a project, and once I get started and begin building the momentum, I have a hard time stopping. It feels so good to see the progress; I don't mind setting aside more time.

Let me share an example with you. My computer was nearing the end of its life, so my husband purchased a new one for me. The new one arrived and sat on the floor of my office for nearly a month. It wasn't for lack of excitement to get it set up; it was because the thought of completely reorganizing my office to make room for the new computer was overwhelming. Finally my husband had had enough. The kids were at school and he had some free time, so he said it was time to get it done. I emptied bookshelves, cleared off my desk, pitched old papers, moved some furniture around and dusted everything. It felt great! Once I got started, my energy was abundant and we got it done. The time passed without a hitch and it felt amazing to have the job completed.

Sometimes you just need to get started and the rest takes care of itself.

SIMPLIFIED HELP

This section is going to give you the answers to questions you may have this week. You may feel as though you hit some stumbling blocks, so hopefully this section will prepare and guide you along the way. Realize that life will always throw you curve balls along the way; it is how you respond to them that makes the difference. So, here are some concerns you may face:

*I cannot stay focused long enough to clean up

So, what happens if your attention span is not very long? Does that mean you are going to ultimately fail at this task? Of course not! It just means you need to prepare yourself before you begin. Maybe you need to spend smaller amounts of time per task. Perhaps you need a partner to motivate you along the way. Possibly you need to create rewards for yourself. It is a great motivator to accomplish a task when you know there is a reward waiting for you. Maybe it's buying something you've wanted for a while. Perhaps it is lunch with a friend. It could be relaxing at a spa. Just remember to set yourself up to succeed. Do whatever it takes to stay on task.

*I am getting overwhelmed with everything I need to de-clutter

Well of course you are! That is precisely why this exercise is so important. Just try to focus on each small task at a time. Looking at the bigger picture will only overwhelm you and stop you in your tracks. Because you have broken down the larger tasks into smaller manageable ones, only focus on one at a time. You need to feel a sense of accomplishment every time you check one area off your list. If the feeling of being overwhelmed is all-consuming, try bringing in some help. Ask a friend to help you. Play some upbeat music while cleaning up. Reward yourself after completing an area. Lighten the load if you need to.

*I can organize everything, but within days it is back to where I started

This is not uncommon! Sometimes it is easy to clean up, but it is the act of staying organized and having a system that is difficult. If organizing does not come naturally to you, you may need to instill some help. Look into hiring a professional organizer. You can research organizers at the national association of professional organizers (www. napo.net) website. Otherwise, research ways you can stay organized. Go to your local office store and ask for their advice. Ask friends how they organize their home and office. Do not give in to the feeling that you can't do it. Push forward to find your own answers!

Get to work! Use this week as an opportunity to clean up what is standing in your way. Focus on one area at a time and before you realize it, you will have an organized space. This space in your life is crucial in preparing you for the larger tasks ahead. These exercises may take a week, they may take a month. It does not really matter. What matters is that you are in action mode. Just the act of "cleaning" up will make space for what really matters to you, whether that is attracting relationships or becoming more productive. Enjoy this process and pat yourself on the back when you complete the tasks at hand.

SIMPLIFIED AFFIRMATIONS

Feel free to use any of these affirmations throughout the week. Saying them out loud will begin to attract them to you. Also say them in the present tense, as if you already have them.

"I am organized and creating healthy space in my life"

"I am attracting people into my life who are helping me create healthy environments"

"It feels great letting go of things that are not necessary in my life anymore. By letting go of these things, I am attracting more enriching and positive items into my life"

Feel free to write down your own affirmations. After you write them down, try to say them on a daily basis.

_____

_____

_____

_____

_____

Week 2

Be in the Moment

I myself have become so preoccupied with the daily tasks of being a mom, running a business, taking care of the home and organizing the meals, that I often lose touch with the here and now. There have been times when I am playing with my children- blowing bubbles on a beautiful spring day- when I'm simultaneously planning the many other things I have on my never-ending to-do list. By the time I have realized this, I've lost the moment. It is forever gone.

Time goes by so quickly, and in a flash the many moments that make up one's life have passed. There will always be work to do, chores to finish, deadlines and responsibilities to live up to. But moments with your children, creating memories with family and friends, will have a much greater impact if you are fully present and aware. Unfortunately, none of us has the capability to look into a glass ball and know what our future holds. So, be conscious of the moment you are in, breathe it in and savor the experiences for what they are.

Growing up, my mother would tell us a story that we called "the strawberry story." This strawberry story had a profound affect on our family for many years. It goes as follows: there was a Buddhist monk who was running from a tiger. He barely made it to the edge of a cliff when he spotted a vine dangling over the edge. He quickly scampered down the vine just as the tiger got to him. Halfway down the vine, he looked down and, sure enough, there was another tiger waiting for him, mouth watering. He looked back up and the first tiger was staring down at him. At the same time, he noticed two small mice, slowly nibbling away at his vine. Just then, he saw a strawberry patch growing vertically on the cliff right next to him. In it was the largest strawberry he ever saw. He plucked it and ate it. It truly was the most delicious strawberry he ever tasted.

The story is a parable for life. It seems there is always a tiger chasing you, a tiger just waiting in ambush for you and something gnawing away at your life line. If, in spite of this, you can still find and enjoy your strawberry each day, you are truly living. By picking a strawberry every day, and by this I mean staying in the moment, you will lead a much richer life than most people.

I want you to shift your awareness this week. I want you to live your life like there is only today. Be in the moment, no matter what task you are completing. *I had a client Norma who practiced this exercise and she said it truly changed her life. Norma was so consumed with the "next" activity, or the "next" chore, that she completely missed the moments that were making up her life. When she started paying attention to her children (really paying attention), her kids' demeanor completely changed. They began behaving better, there were fewer fights, they obeyed more, and the family dynamic improved. All of this came to pass because she lived more in the moment and got back in the game of life.* I myself have noticed times when I was multitasking to a degree that I was missing the important elements of my life. Keep in mind what is most important to you, and then make sure to be present for these things.

Tips for the Week

1. Out of sight...out of mind

This week try to be fully aware of each moment. Keep work at the workplace, and when you are home, really enjoy the time with your loved ones. Play just for the sake of playing. Realize that work will get done during designated hours at the office. Schedule time to just "be" and try to put work issues and concerns out of your mind, even if for just a short moment.

2. Be in the moment

Say the phrase "be in the moment" when you find yourself drifting to other things. When playing with your children, enjoying alone time with your spouse, or having lunch with a friend, just be, and relish what you are doing in that moment. The more you practice this, the more natural it will become in your life. Like anything, you are changing a behavior. It takes time and patience, so try not to get frustrated. Just do your best.

3. Have fun!

Being in the moment will take on a life of its own. What is the point of all of this if you are not having fun and enjoying yourself? The more you balance work and play, the more productive and aware you will become in everything you do.

Work does not need to consume your every thought, nor does being carefree and neglecting responsibilities. Just remember, it is ok to compartmentalize different parts of your life. Have fun and work hard! Because my children are young, I have a constant reminder of how precious time is and how quickly it goes. When my life is near the end, I will cherish the memories and time spent with loved ones. Just try to be aware of how you are spending your time. This awareness will keep you grounded in the things that truly matter.

SIMPLIFIED HELP

* I try to be in the moment, I but cannot focus

OK, so you have tried this exercise, but you cannot get all the clutter out of your head? Instead of trying this cold turkey, take small steps. Can you begin by focusing your mind on small periods of time? Look at your calendar and determine when you will practice the art of being in the moment. Are you attending one of your child's soccer games this week? Maybe commit to enjoying the game, free from any gadgets such as your cell phone or blackberry. This is about starting small and working up to the bigger tasks. Focus a little at a time and then the difficulty will lessen over time.

* My plate is too full to be in the moment

This is exactly why you need to practice this! If you are going in so many different directions, that you are not able to fully enjoy any of them, what is the point? I want you to take a good hard look at how you are spending your time. Are you consciously choosing how you are spending your time? Can you let go of some obligations that do not have as much meaning to you? If you can lessen your load, you will ultimately enjoy your life on a richer level. Having a full plate is great if you can handle it, but if it is depleting you and your time, you need to do something about it.

*Have fun? I do not even know where to begin

One of the exercises this week is to have fun. Have you forgotten how to have fun and create some playtime? I know from personal experience how easy it is to get consumed with "life."

If you are so wrapped up in work, in obligations, in doing for others, that you have forgotten how to have fun, it is time to stop and look deeper. Take some time to remember your past and reflect on what brought you joy. Do you love tapping into your creativity? Do you enjoy the great outdoors? Do you love reading a good book? Do you miss time with friends? Make a list of all the things that put a smile on your face and then start putting them to action.

Now it is time to re-engage in the game of life. Just remember when you are feeling overly consumed with work or obligations, take a step back and live your life in the moment by enjoying the simple things. Practice and commitment to live your life to the fullest will keep you motivated and enthused to keep going. Good luck!

SIMPLIFIED AFFIRMATIONS

"I am living my life in the moment"

"Being in the moment is allowing me to see the beauty all around me"

"I am grounded and centered in what really matters"

"Every day I am able to enjoy the little things and feel joy and peace"

Say these affirmations daily as a means to create them with intention.

Week 3

Closure is needed before new opportunities

The simple act of closing one door so you can open another is not a myth. I want you to visualize an actual doorway with you standing in the middle. You have one foot inside the door with one foot outside the door. You physically cannot be in and out at the same time. A good example is when people are puzzled as to why they have one failed relationship after another. You want to meet someone, even though you have not processed and moved on from your previous relationship. You then wonder why you cannot create a healthy partnership with someone new. You need to categorize the past in the past so that you are free to move on to the next chapter in your life.

What does this tell you? If you truly want to move forward in relationships, in your career, or in any other area of your life, you need to decide on what side of the door you want to stand. Remember that things in your past are there for a reason-it was either not meant to be or it was the wrong time. Either way, you have a choice to make. Continue living in the past, or open yourself up to the possibilities the future holds for you.

Let me share my own life experience with this model. I did not date very seriously prior to meeting my husband, because I always knew fairly early on that the men I dated were not life companions. I did meet one person that I dated on and off for around six months. This for me was a world record, for most men were lucky to make it to the third or fourth date. We eventually parted ways, and at the time I was heartbroken. This was my first lasting relationship and it was difficult to let it go. Looking back, it was not meant to be. The bigger plan was to cross paths with my now husband and create a life together. If I had continued to compare future men with my ex-boyfriend, I would still be single and looking. Some part of me realized I needed to stand tall and move on. I knew I deserved better and I luckily had the know-how to move on.

A client named Sarah was having an extremely difficult time letting go of a past relationship. The couple broke up nearly two years prior, and she was still holding on to the hope that they would get back together. After working together for a couple of months, she came to the realization that she was allowing an unrealistic expectation to control her every thought. She was so consumed with the past that in no way was she able to embrace the present or future. She was able to put some closure on the relationship and begin her journey forward. By closing the door to the past, she was finally free to live her life on her terms.

I share this story for several reasons. First, be true to yourself above all else. Know that you deserve only the best, no matter what the circumstances, and don't ever settle for less. And lastly, take note of where in your life you are standing in the doorway. Choose now to either step out or stay in, and then be at peace with your decision.

Tips for the Week

1. Ask yourself questions

You first need to determine why you are holding onto certain memories and periods of your life. Is what you are holding onto helping you move on with your life or holding you back? What will realistically happen if you let this go? What are the potential gains from letting this go? Also ask yourself what you are gaining by holding on to the past.

2. Think about the pros and cons

Once you have answered the first set of questions, you need to dig a little deeper. What are the pros from leaving the past in the past? What fears arise as to why you have not been able to move forward? What are the cons from continuously diving into your past? Don't settle for superficial answers. Dig until you are satisfied with the answers.

3. Create a plan

Now that you have committed to moving forward, you need a plan to support you. What resources and support can you create to help you stay on track and focused? Know what your obstacles will be and create ways to overcome them. Surround yourself with individuals who will hold you accountable. Also, keep in mind what you will be gaining by staying on course. Creating a plan is very empowering because it gives you your power back. You are not a victim of past circumstances; you are now in control of your future and your destiny.

Remember, when you close one door, you are allowing other doors to open and opportunities to present themselves to you. Living in the past is just that- the past. If you want to embrace the future, you need to open yourself up to it. Have faith in the bigger picture and trust that things happen for reasons that at the time may or may not make sense to you.

SIMPLIFIED HELP

*I try closing the door, but it keeps opening

Some of you may feel as though you close the door on a chapter in your life, and then it reopens all on its own. There may be times that the door cracks open every now and then. Don't beat yourself up over it. If you continue to focus on the future and moving forward little by little, then the door will slowly remain closed on its own. Just maintain your integrity, keep a positive attitude, and know that you will be ok. Remember that doors do not open on their own; it takes someone to open or shut them. Acknowledge that you have the power to do either one.

*I do not have the strength to step on the other side

You absolutely have the strength! Humans are so much stronger and more resilient than we give ourselves credit for. We just don't give ourselves the opportunity to tap into this strength. Too many give up way before that strength would have kicked in. Even if you are unfamiliar with this inner strength, please have faith that it is there somewhere. Maybe it just needs to be dusted off a bit. Start small and work your way up. When my mother passed away I never thought I would have the strength to move on with my life. I would have loved to have stayed inside my room and not venture outward, but that is not what she would have wanted. She was so full of life that it would have been an insult not to live my life to the fullest.

SIMPLIFIED AFFIRMATIONS

"I have an inner strength that will always guide and protect me"

"I am surrounded by people who will help me move forward in my life"

"I trust that my inner compass will lead me in the right direction"

"I am supported completely when leaving the past in the past"

"I am ready to embark on my future with excitement"

Keep in mind that you do not need to cross through ten doors at once. Pick one door at a time and walk through it. Every door you step through will give you the confidence to walk through more. Like anything in life, breaking down large tasks into smaller ones will make it feel more approachable. You just need to acknowledge why you have not been able to move forward from your past. What is holding you back? If you need help, then absolutely seek it out. We all reminisce about the past, but if your reminiscing is all-consuming, then you need to determine what you can do to slowly move forward with your life. Have a good week.

Week 4

Don't wait, make the first move!

When my son began kindergarten, it was a huge step in his little life. Of course he was anxious, I was anxious, my husband was anxious. Like any mom, I wanted to do whatever I could to create a smooth and comfortable transition for him. I thought it would make such a huge difference if my son was able to meet some kids in his class prior to the first day of school. Of course the school was too busy to prepare something like this, so I took it upon myself to do something. I am not the type of person to wait for someone else to clear a trail, I'm happy to take the initiative myself. So, I called the principal and shared my idea of hosting an informal gathering at my home, and she gave me an enthusiastic thumbs up. Long story short, I had about fifteen children and their mothers at my home and we all had a great time. The kids made instant friends, and it gave the mom's an opportunity to get to know each other as well. The kids were a lot less nervous and apprehensive about starting a new school. They saw familiar faces and it made the transition go much smoother.

There will be many times in your own life when you feel the need to create your own path. It is much easier to stay in the background and hope someone else will make the first move. *I had a client, Donna, who was beginning the dating scene after a lengthy marriage had fallen apart. She was new to the rules of dating and was a bit hesitant to get out there. Once we built her esteem up a bit and she was feeling better about herself and what she had to offer, she was ready to embark on the journey. She began to date, but kept talking about this gentleman that she worked with. She was friendly with him at work and was always intrigued by him. However, she was nervous to make the first move and was more comfortable waiting for him to approach her. After discussing the pros and cons of waiting, possibly for quite some time, she was ready to take the risk. She decided to ask him to coffee and see where it went from there. To her amazement, not only did he say yes, but he was extremely flattered and happy that she approached him first. He was hesitant to ask her out at work, for he didn't want to make her feel uncomfortable in any way if she was not interested. To make my point, had she waited on the sidelines, she might still be waiting. Sometimes taking risks is what keeps us alive and engaged in the game of life. And, yes, the two of them are still happily dating to this day.*

This week's focus is about creating your own trail- dancing to your own tune. The people who truly succeed in life are the ones who make things happen for themselves. They don't wait for life to happen to them, they create it! So take some time to examine where in your own life you are holding back. Getting out of your comfort zone is where you will experience the most gratifying of times. Once you move past the fear and trepidation, you will stand taller and more confident in who you are and what you want.

ACTION STEPS FOR THE WEEK:

1. What are you waiting for?

Where in your life are you holding back? Are there specific situations where you are waiting for someone else to make the first move? Why give everyone else the power that you can harness yourself? Do you have ideas at work? Do you want to cultivate a relationship with someone new? Would you like to make amends with someone, although you have been waiting for them to make the first move? Journal what comes to mind.

_____

_____

_____

_____

_____

_____

_____

2. Take steps

Now that you have a detailed list in front of you, take a good hard look at it. Are there situations that you would be willing to take a risk? Are there things you have been going back and forth on? Life is about taking risks and being willing to fall every now and then. Most of the time we brainstorm in our minds a scenario and outcome that is unrealistic. We assume the worst, therefore holding ourselves back before giving it a try. All I ask of you this week is to explore outside of your comfort zone and begin to move forward in your life.

3. Leader vs follower

Do you want to be a leader or a follower in your life? If you are comfortable following the lead of others, then that is great. If, however, you are ready to step up to the plate and direct your own life, then there is no better time than the present. Begin with small risks, build up your confidence muscle a bit, and then explore the larger issues in your life. Where in your life can you take small risks first? By starting small, you will gain confidence as you go, thus giving you the push to do more.

SIMPLIFIED HELP

*I am just not a born leader

This exercise is not about making you something you are not. Some people are born leaders and others are comfortable in the background. What I would like for you is to not be shy and content with areas of your life where you would like to see change. You can spend a lot of time waiting for others to make it "right," or you can take control of your life and be proactive. If you do not naturally lead, then do what feels comfortable. Just pushing the boundaries a bit and stepping outside your comfort zone will promote growth.

*I have failed in the past, so why bother?

Even the best of us have failed and experienced disappointment. If you have tried to be a leader and you've been disappointed, are you ok with throwing in the towel? The most successful people in the world have failed and failed again. What makes them different is the ability to keep going even when the going gets tough. They know that failure is an opportunity to grow and build character; they do not see it as a setback. I guarantee if you try and try again, eventually things will fall into place. Do not ever be satisfied with your life just happening to you; choose the course you are going to take.

So, back to the story of my son and kindergarten. He survived the first year of school and I am genuinely able to pat myself on the back for everything I did. I gave him the opportunity to get to know the children in his class, and then I left it up to him to cultivate the friendships. I set up play dates, I arranged parties for the holidays, I volunteered many times in the classroom and all in all I was an engaged parent. I could have sat on the sidelines and left it up to my child to navigate and figure things out on his own. Or, I could set up the environment at his comfort level, and let him do his thing at his own pace. He figured it out and is completely ready to do it again next year. Just take a look at your own life and decide where you can make the first move!

SIMPLIFIED AFFIRMATIONS

"I always have the strength and guidance to move forward in my life"

"I am confident in my abilities to make decisions and stick to them"

"I have released the fear of being proactive in my own life"

"I am in control of my destiny"

Say these affirmations daily or create your own. Remember the act of affirming your desires will begin to manifest them.

Week 5

Embrace gratitude in your life

How often do you truly express gratitude for everything you have in your life? Do you do it solely during the holidays when it is expected? Do you do it when tragedies occur and you feel obligated to do this? It is easy to get preoccupied with life's details that you simply put gratitude out of your mind. Between work, family, and responsibilities, it makes sense that expressing gratitude is not at the top of your to-do list. What if I told you the sheer act of expressing gratitude sends an invisible signal to the Universe to send you more things to be grateful for? Would you then put some time into this? It would be easy to look at people less fortunate and then give thanks for all you have, for they would trade lives with you in a split second. Why not make gratitude part of your daily ritual? Embracing gratitude not only keeps you focused on the now, but it makes you appreciative of all you *do* have in your life. Instead of wasting energy complaining about what you *don't* have, spend the same energy on what *is* currently in your life that you are appreciative for.

A client, Susan, who I worked with spent much time and energy focused on what was not working in her life. She complained about her job even though it was extremely lucrative and affording her many luxuries. She complained about her lack of quality friends even though she had several genuine friends that stood by her through thick and thin. She complained about being single even though she enjoyed traveling with girlfriends and spending quiet time in her beautiful home. She somehow tuned out all the good that surrounded her and only noticed the things that were lacking. Very quickly after beginning our work together Susan began to broaden her ways of looking at her life. She realized she did have so much to be grateful for and she enjoyed how she felt when she focused on the positive. She realized by focusing on all she had to be grateful for, she was some how attracting more of that to her.

If I asked you right now what you are grateful for, what would you say? Would you hesitate? Would you start to list things left and right? No matter where you are in your life, there is always something to be grateful for. If you just lost a job, can you be grateful that you have your health? If your health is deteriorating, can you be grateful for your friends and family that are supporting you? If you are single and unhappy, can you be grateful for your freedom and ability to start fresh?

Yes, I am an eternal optimist, but I have also had my fair share of disappointments and heart aches. Losing my mother was the most difficult experience I ever had to survive, but somehow I was able to focus one day at a time. I understand when you are immersed in the moment, it is difficult to feel grateful for anything in your life. Just the act of expressing gratitude will lift your spirits and put things in perspective.

John was having difficulty feeling grateful for all he had in his life. He was going through a difficult divorce; he was unhappy at work; he was living a sedentary lifestyle and he just wasn't engaged in life anymore. I wasn't about to ask him what he was grateful for when we first began working together. That would have been counterproductive. However, after working on lifting his self esteem, bringing activity back into his life, and seeking new employment, was he able to talk about it. He then realized he had a lot to be grateful for. He had a beautiful home and was raising healthy and well-adjusted children. He was grateful to find work he was passionate about, and most importantly he was grateful for his friends that stuck by him through a very difficult time.

If you find yourself complaining more than normal, bring some gratitude back into your life. The more appreciative you are, the more you attract that positive flow into your life. If you are having a hard time accepting this concept, give it a try. Use this week as an experiment in expressing gratitude, and see if it changes your life and more importantly if it elevates your mood.

ACTION STEPS FOR THE WEEK

1. Keep a gratitude journal

Purchase a journal this week to record what you are grateful for. Every evening write down five things you were grateful for that day. This helps develop your awareness for being in the moment. If you are not much of a writer, feel free to express your gratefulness in other ways. Maybe say them to yourself before bed. Either way, make this ritual a part of your day. It is also important not to write down the same things every evening. You will probably start this journal with the bigger items, such as being grateful for your home, your health, your friends and family. As the days go on, you will need to search a little deeper. Maybe you were grateful for the beautiful sunset you witnessed. Or, you were grateful that a complete stranger smiled and made your day. Just have fun with this journal and see what you come up with.

2. Smell the roses

As hectic as your life may seem, take a moment every day to smell the roses. Look for the simple things every day that put a smile on your face, and really embrace the feeling it brings you. Life is made up of all the "little moments." Some examples may be a smile from a stranger, a hug from a friend, an unexpected compliment, or a phone call from an old friend. Smelling the roses is a reminder of the miracle of life. It will help ground you amidst all the stressors.

3. Communicate your feelings

Make a commitment this week to tell the people in your life how you feel about them. Don't wait until tomorrow; don't wait for a later date, you never know what tomorrow will bring. Show your appreciation now. This exercise keeps you focused in the moment, helping you enjoy the here and now. How do you feel when others express their feelings to you? Does it feel good? Is it an emotional boost? Know that you have the power to light up someone else's day. A simple statement could be exactly what they needed at that moment.

When I am feeling out of sorts, I take the time to express everything I am grateful for. Even if I say them to myself, it puts me in a better mood and lifts my spirits. A friend of mine asked me to sign up for a triathlon with her. Keep in mind, I was not an overachieving athlete in any way, so I knew it would be a huge accomplishment. Knowing that I had to swim in an open water lake pushed me into do or die mode. I was never a swimmer, and when I began to train I could barely swim one lap without hyperventilating. I had my work cut out for me. The reason I am sharing this story is because the more I swam, the more I loved the experience. Being in the water, with absolutely no outside distractions, became meditative for me. I used the opportunity to say everything I was grateful for, and state my positive affirmations as well. I looked forward to swimming and I felt so much better the rest of the day.

SIMPLIFIED HELP

* I feel like I have nothing to be grateful for

Just the fact that you are reading this book right now means you have your eyesight. There are many individuals that would give anything to see the world around them. This is just one example, but I guarantee there are many more. Taking a step back from what is missing in your life, can you focus on a couple of areas that you are grateful for? Are there some positives that stand out? Just refocus your energy on what *is* working in your life, not what is **not** working.

*It is hard to smell the roses when I am constantly on the run

I know firsthand how difficult it can feel when your life is constantly on the go. I also know how crucial it is to stop every now and then. When I begin to feel frazzled, I know it is time to take a break and just breathe. Learn the signals and then have activities or ideas that you can engage in to ground you and put things in perspective. Maybe it is grabbing a coffee with a friend, or visiting your local botanic garden. It could be getting a massage or taking a nice long walk. Just know what works for you and commit to doing it when the chaos begins to surround you.

SIMPLIFIED AFFIRMATIONS

"I am grateful that I am attracting positive and enriching people into my life"

"I am grateful for what I do have in my life, and I am constantly attracting light energy to myself"

"I am grateful that people are coming into my life to help me on my journey"

"I am grateful that I have the tools and insight to live the best life possible"

Feel free to say the above affirmations on a daily basis, or create your own that feel good and empowering. Use the space below to write what comes to mind.

_____

_____

_____

_____

_____

_____

_____

_____

_____

Just so you know, I did finish the triathlon, and I did not need to be rescued from the lake either. It was a wonderful experience that I would highly recommend. I continue to swim to this day, and I love the quiet time and peacefulness of it all. Sometimes venturing out and trying new things is just what the body and soul needs. So, for this week, practice the art of expressing gratitude. Remember there is no right or wrong way to do this, just do what feels right.

Week 6

Fear Can Be Converted to Freedom

I know from first hand experience how easy it is to allow fear to control the choices you make in life; fear of success, fear of failure, fear of the unknown or the known. It is an easy way out and comfortable to stay where you are in life. Fear is a form of protection, but when it dictates the choices you make in life, it can hinder your growth. How often in your life did you have the desire to do something but then that nervous voice in your head talked you out of it? You know that voice, the one that doubts your abilities and tries to keep you from venturing out and taking risks.

A client of mine, Barb, was at the point in her career where she was desperately seeking a change. She was ready to do something else, but her fear of financial distress and possible failure held her back. Her fear was real to an extent, but she had two choices ahead of her. She could both give in to the fear and stay where she was, or she could formulate a plan and be willing to take the risks involved.

After discussing the pros and cons of staying where she was, and the pros and cons of starting her own company, it was clear what she wanted to do. She realized her current job was never going to provide what it was she was looking for, and she needed to follow her passions. By detailing a very specific blue print for her, and breaking down her long term goal into manageable baby steps, she felt a sigh of relief. She picked a date that she would give notice to her current employer, and then she began the process of venturing forward with her new idea.

Have you ever had a specific fear that continued to show itself from time to time? Maybe yours was a fear of commitment. Because this fear was so great, you had a tendency to sabotage every relationship that came your way. How would it feel to embrace the fear wholeheartedly and move past it? Would it feel refreshing and empowering? When you are able to push past a fear, you not only grow as a person but you open yourself up to opportunities that might not have been presented to you in the past. Turning your fear into freedom allows you to live your life from purpose and vision. This in turn allows you to take control of your life, not allowing fear to control the decisions you make and the paths you follow.

Once Barb faced her fears of failure and financial distress, she was able to put things in perspective. She always achieved things in her life, so why would this be any different? She realized that most of her fears were blown way out of proportion. She was looking at the worst case scenario and neglecting to focus on her strengths and how she would succeed. She realized the risks she was going to take would far surpass staying where she was and being unhappy. She needed to bring life back into her otherwise disheartening existence. Once she secured the date to leave her current employer, everything else fell into place. She realized that her fear was valid to an extent, but it did not need to hold her back any longer. She felt a huge sense of relief knowing that she was finally following her dream. She felt empowered and strong in her venture. As the date quickly approached, her fears dissipated and excitement took over. Currently she is extremely happy in all elements of her life and her business is thriving. Barb realized that the fear she held onto for so long had stopped her in evolving in many other areas of her life. She is grateful every day for finding the strength to move forward and follow her heart.

Fear is a normal part of existence; there is no getting around it. However, when it becomes the compass that guides your decisions, it is time to make a change. By surrounding yourself by people and resources to help you succeed, you will thrive no matter what the outcome. Sometimes it is just a matter of taking your power back by researching your options and detailing a plan. I remember early in my career an organization asked me to be a keynote speaker at one of their events. There would have been several hundred people, and my initial instinct was total fear that I would make a fool of myself. I told them I would check my calendar and get back to them. I knew the easy and safe choice would be to say no. I also knew that by giving in to the fear, I would never grow or evolve. So, I accepted their offer and was absolutely petrified for months. However, because I planned my speech and practiced hundreds of times, I felt comfortable when the day came. Once I was on the stage speaking from my heart, the nervousness subsided and I had an absolutely wonderful time. Had I given in to the fear, I would have been disappointed in myself. I needed to break through the initial fear of speaking so that I could fine tune my craft and do more speaking engagements. This week will give you the opportunity to clarify your own fears and you will gain the tools to move past them.

ACTION STEPS FOR THE WEEK

1. List your fears

Make a list of all of your current fears. Some examples may be fear of a new job, fear of committing in a relationship, fear of confronting a friend, or fear of financial distress. Once you have this master list, you need to take it to the next step. How are these current fears holding you back from moving forward in your life? Let us assume one of your fears is committing in a relationship. How is your lack of commitment holding you back? Are you unable to enjoy all the benefits of being in a committed relationship? Are you holding back the possibility of starting a family? Make this list and then dig a little deeper.

2. Detail scenarios

Choose one fear at a time. Write down what your life will look like if you continue to allow your fear to hold you back. Now write down what your life may potentially look like if you face the fear head on and move past it. Which path looks more promising? Which path creates growth? This is not a trick question, just answer it honestly. It is absolutely your choice to play it safe and stay within your comfort zone. I just want to make sure that you are ok with that choice. If you know that it is time to tap in to your inner strength, then I give you permission to do so.

3. Tap into resources

Having resources and support is crucial when facing your fears. Now is the time to do some research. Most of the time, people procrastinate because they don't know the next step or where to turn. Alleviate this problem by educating yourself and getting answers. Along with this, it is important to surround yourself by individuals who support your growth. Maybe you need to work with a financial advisor to feel prepared. Possibly you need to hire a life coach to help create a blueprint for your life. Maybe it is talking to human resources about a problem you are having at work. Just know that it is ok to ask for help when needed.

Try not to rush through this section of the book. Facing your fears is something that may take a couple weeks, or it may take several months. As long as you are moving in a forward direction, then go at your own pace. Even though I do this for a living, I am constantly facing my own fears. Situations will pop up in my own life that force me to tap into my own inner strength. That is what life is all about- opportunities presenting themselves to help you grow and evolve.

SIMPLIFIED HELP

*My fears are overwhelming

If you feel your fears are too big to tackle on your own, then bring on some help. There is nothing wrong with supporting yourself to succeed. It is acknowledging that you are stuck in fear that will begin to push you forward. Seek out a therapist. Hire a life coach. Join a support group. Just the act of discussing your fears and not bottling them up will be a huge step in the right direction.

*My fears are very valid

If your fears are valid and therefore you are hesitant to move past them, you still have some options. Let's take for example you fear leaving a job that would put you into financial distress. Of course this is a valid fear and a fear that you should listen to. It doesn't mean you can't leave the job ever, it just means that you need to do a bit more research and planning. Maybe you need to put away six months of expenses before you leave. Possibly it means researching other jobs and fine tuning your resume. If you prepare and feel confident in a specific plan of action, your fears will generally dissipate.

* I prefer to stay in my comfort zone

Let me be very clear here. You do not need to face your fears if you choose not to. There is no rule book that says you are failing if you stay safe. This is completely your choice and yours alone. However, some people like to feel safe, but they also know it is important for their growth to push the boundaries from time to time. They just go at a pace that works for them. So, if you are content with staying where you are, then keep doing just that. If, however, you are content but willing to venture out a bit, then I support you to do that as well.

SIMPLIFIED AFFIRMATIONS

"I am always protected when facing my fears"

"I believe in myself and my abilities"

"Fear will no longer define my life and who I am"

"I am capable of moving past my own limitations"

"I am completely supported"

Remember to take your time when processing through this week's assignments. Just the fact that you are reading this book is a huge step in the right direction. Just know that I support your growth and believe in you 100%. Living in fear is no way to live. Live from love and light and feel the difference. Even by tackling just one fear at a time, this will allow you to feel more comfortable with the process. Keep up the good work so you can continue moving forward.

Week 7

Get your own needs met first

We all have needs in life, and when these needs are fulfilled we feel complete and whole. Some of us need to feel loved. Some need to be heard. Some need freedom to express and explore. Unfortunately, most people look outside themselves to fill these needs. *Let me give you an example from a client of mine named Joyce. Joyce was a beautiful woman in her mid-thirties, but she didn't have the best childhood. She never received praise and unconditional love from her father and therefore she always looked to other men to fill that void. She lacked self confidence and she did not feel very worthy of being treated kindly by men. Because of this need to feel loved and accepted, and more importantly, the fact that she did not love herself first, she always attracted the wrong guy. Until she realized that loving and nurturing herself was the most important first step, she continued the cycle she was on. Most people don't realize that they can fulfill their own needs first, before looking to others to do it for them. How would it feel to take the burden off others while providing it yourself? Then you would naturally attract people into your life that would respect and honor your needs. No one wants to feel forced to fill a need that you have. They would rather offer it genuinely and in their own way.*

Women generally have guilt associated with putting their needs at the top of their priority list. I have been guilty of this in the past myself, so I know the importance of honoring this ability. Unfortunately, over time we get so comfortable not meeting our own needs that we naturally assume someone else should do it for us. This is when you get into trouble. When you *expect* someone to fill a need, you will never be happy or satisfied. It is important to recognize when you are going down this path so that you can change course. Early in my marriage, I went through a period where I expected my husband to focus more on romance. Even when he made the effort, I would find something to be upset about. I realized that it was simply because I was feeling insecure and I was looking to him to make me feel better. Do you think it worked? Temporarily, but not long-term. I needed to start nurturing myself and boost my own self confidence. I was able to fill my own void without expecting him to do it for me. I learned an invaluable lesson. Never underestimate the power of doing what it takes to feel better. If you are insecure with your body, work with a trainer or find a work out buddy. If you lack communication skills, sign up for an improv class or work with a coach. Fill your own needs and you will have so much more to offer all those around you. Get rid of the guilt!

This concept does not exclusively apply to women. *I worked with a gentleman named Jerry who struggled with this concept. He was a top executive at a major telecommunications firm. He was powerful in his own right and got used to being in this position. He definitely had a need for power and control and he needed others to validate this for him. Unfortunately, he was unable to draw a line between work and family. Because of his need for power, he expected the same form of treatment from his wife and kids. Obviously this did not go over well. Once he realized this fundamental need and the reason he had it in the first place, he was able to make some changes. He was able to fill this need in a more positive and productive way at work and not carry it home. Sometimes it just takes a bit of detective work in order to move forward in your life.*

This week I would like you to spend some time clarifying for yourself what your own needs are. What are the needs that guide you in your life? What do you naturally gravitate toward? Peeling away these layers will help you unveil the real reasons you act certain ways. If you always get bored and feel antsy after being somewhere for a set amount of time, one of your primal needs may be adventure and challenge. If you have a tendency to have relationship after relationship, possibly with married men or women, you may have a primal need to feel excitement and feel wanted. Obviously, there are healthier ways to get this need met, but that is another book in entirety. Take a break, get out your notebook and get to work. This chapter will give you an opportunity to identify patterns and possibly break some unhealthy ones.

ACTION STEPS FOR THE WEEK

1. What are your needs?

Make a detailed list of all of your needs. Some examples may be safety, joy, abundance, control, acceptance or love. Your needs are what you feel you cannot live without. These needs guide all of your decisions and actions in your life. Let's say you have a need for safety and comfort. You need to feel safe. Because of this need, you may have difficulty taking risks and moving outside your comfort zone. Just realizing this need may help you begin to move forward and take baby steps. Taking small risks will allow you to grow and open opportunities for yourself that might not have existed otherwise. Many people do not take the time to explore what their needs are, and therefore they wonder why they act certain ways and react under certain circumstances. Take the time this week.

2. Narrow the list

From the list you made above, I want you to narrow it down to your top five needs. I want you then to take it one step further. Narrow this list to your top three. This shows your three most important core needs. These needs are your excuse behind your behaviors. What do I mean by that? Let's say one of your core needs is creativity. You need to have creativity in your life or you feel empty and unfulfilled. Many of the choices you make in life revolve around this need. Let's say you have a well paying job, but it is very cyclical day in and day out. There is not much variety and there are not many opportunities to bring a creative element to the table. Therefore you are miserable and unhappy most of the time. You assume there is something wrong with you for being dissatisfied, instead of realizing it is just not a good fit. An ideal profession would be one that involves imagination and creativity. Look at this list and then look at your life.

3. Commit to act

From this list of three needs, I want you to focus on fulfilling one need per week. If your first need is love, pick five loving acts you can do for yourself this week. You can get a massage, meet a friend for lunch, go for a walk, take a hot bath, read a great book or commit to many other nurturing acts. See how it feels to be consistent with your behavior. Instead of looking to others to fill the void, fill your own needs. It is always much more powerful when we take ownership for feeling a certain way. By meeting your own needs, you can fully enjoy when someone else nurtures them as well. Then it won't be expected, but appreciated. It is always the action behind the desires that are missing. So, this week it is about acting upon your core needs. Be proactive and forward moving.

One of my core needs is laughter and joy. Observing my mother's illnesses growing up, I realized at a very young age how important it was to find joy and laughter in the everyday ups and downs. Life was too important and sacred to be taken so seriously. My mom laughed every day, the deep belly-hurt laughs that were so contagious. Because this is one of my core needs, I don't feel good when I go a period of time without having fun. I then re-focus on the basics and find joy in the simple things. This keeps me happy and grounded on what really matters. So, take some time to clarify what matters the most to you, and then bring it into your life on a daily basis.

SIMPLIFIED HELP

*I feel guilty focusing on my own needs

I know many of you reading this book are natural caregivers. I myself feel drawn to taking care of others. It becomes a problem, however, when you neglect yourself in the process. Why do you feel guilty? What is so wrong with nurturing your needs? Maybe you are just used to putting yourself last, so this is very foreign to you. That's ok. I don't want you to skip over this step. It just means you need to go at your own pace. I guarantee you will feel stronger and more confident if you nurture your needs and tend to them.

*I've always looked to others to "complete" me

If you've created a pattern of looking to others to fulfill your needs, it does not mean you are stuck in this pattern for the rest of your life. Just because you are used to doing something one way, doesn't mean there are not three other ways to go about it. I want you to regain your power and nurture your needs, so you never again expect someone to do it for you. You have to trust me on this one. Just venture out and know that you are supported the whole time.

* I can't seem to narrow down my needs

You've read everything for this week's assignment, and you are completely stuck. Please know that I completely understand how difficult some of these exercises are. Most of us don't take the time to slow down enough in life to answer deeper questions on who we are. Just clarify for yourself what needs strike a chord with you. Here are some examples:

*Family	*Belonging	*Fun	*Honesty	*Trust
*Success	*Peace	*Love	*Health	*Structure
*Safety	*Abundance	*Support	*Space	*Control

Take your time and do your best. Sometimes you just need to take a break so that you can come back at a later date and have a different perspective. Good luck!

SIMPLIFIED AFFIRMATIONS

"My needs are always met and provided for"

"I am worth nurturing my needs"

"I know that by nurturing my own needs, I will always have more to give to others"

"I do not need anyone to fill my needs for me, my needs are always provided for"

Let me just say that I am proud of you for all of your work up to this point in the book. No matter how far you have come, or how many chapters you have tackled, pat yourself on the back for the dedication and willingness to improve your life. This week gave you the opportunity to see why you behave certain ways. You should realize that your core needs propel you to experience life through a specific set of glasses. There is no right or wrong, it just is. Good job and keep the positive momentum going.

Week 8

Handle stress with ease

With everything going on in the world around us, from wars to the economy, to gas prices, it is difficult not to be affected. How stressed are you in your own life right now? I try not to get caught up in the magnitude of everything. I have compassion and try to do what I can to make the world a better place, but I do not focus on it all the time. As frightening as things can feel at times, I choose to focus on the blessings and joys in my life. I know things will bounce back, so stressing about them will not change the fact. Do you sometimes feel you are on edge more than normal? Do you feel less capable of handling life's stressors? Your body's response to stress can have serious consequences, both on a physical and emotional level. There have been numerous studies of the body's negative reaction to stress. Reactions can vary from heightened allergies, to heart disease and depression. I am sure everyone reading this book can think of someone in their life that is a high-stress individual. Maybe they seem constantly on edge. Possibly they tend to have a constant stream of health issues. Maybe they seem to attract negative situations into their life. Needless to say, the ongoing stress they carry adds up in a big way.

I once worked with a gentleman that constantly struggled with his inability to cope with stressful situations. On the outside he appeared to have a great life, but internally he was spiraling downward. He worried about everything and never fully enjoyed all the blessings in his life. The stress he put on himself was literally killing him and he knew it. He reached out for help coping with all life's stressors that were presenting themselves to him.

I helped him see his life through a different lens, and slowly he was able to reprogram his negative thoughts and reactions. He learned when he needed to take some time to himself, and he came to value this alone time. He also learned to roll things off his shoulders in a way that he was never able to do. Not everything in the universe revolved around him, and he needed to understand this concept in order to move forward.

I am a go-getter in many forms, so this was a lesson I too needed to learn. I would work myself up until my stress level was oozing every cell in my body. I would take on one too many commitments, feeling like every one was of critical importance, until my body and mind were near collapsing. My husband was great about pointing the obvious out to me, but as usual I had to come to the realization on my own. I needed to find a way of dealing with my stress so that it wouldn't consume me. For me, it was about taking time to myself and honoring my health. Time alone gave me the ability to take a breath and compose my thoughts. It was just stopping long enough to regain my composure and make sure my priorities were in check. It was a mental and emotional break. I also made my health a top priority. Regular exercise became meditative for me, and it helped me cope with everything going on. It was a natural energy boost.

I still have a lot on my plate, between work, kids, activities, and planning meals. I know when the stress piles up I can take a step back and just breathe. I love my life and everything I have going on, but I also know the effects of stress. I've released the guilt of asking for help when it's needed. This week I want you to be conscious of your stress level and take the steps to combat it. Life is stressful, there is no way around it, but there are many ways you can face the stress and keep enjoying your life.

ACTION STEPS FOR THE WEEK:

1. Take time outs

There is no way you can control everything in your life, nor would you want to. But, you do have the ability to bring some calm to stressful situations. When you feel your stress level rising, take a time out. We use this method with our children, but it is just as useful and necessary for adults. This week practice taking some deep breaths, go for a walk, or simply spend some much needed time alone. I have two young children whom I adore, but they know how to raise my stress level on a daily basis. I use time outs for myself often. It just gives me some time to let the emotions go down a notch, and then I am much more able to talk with my children in a constructive way. I guarantee walking away every now and then will improve your life dramatically. Try it this week.

2. Stay healthy

If your body is healthy you will be much better equipped to handle stressful situations. When we feed our body excessive sugar and fatty foods, the immune system is not as capable of fending off illness. This leads to sickness, fatigue, and feeling lousy. Stock up on fruits, vegetables and whole grains. Feeding your body an assortment of healthy foods will help you handle life's ups and downs. I know this seems like an obvious tip, but there are so many individuals who make unhealthy choices. Whether it is a matter of convenience, or they are eating to fill an emotional void, this habit is absolutely no good. If you are not sure what it takes to make healthy choices, ask for help. Work with a dietician or nutritionist, or just ask a friend for some helpful advice. There are always ways you can embrace a healthy lifestyle. This week commit to doing what you can to feed your body foods that give you natural energy.

3. Ask for support

As reported in Psychological Review in July 2000, women live an average of five years longer than men. Why is this you ask? Women are much better at reaching for support when they are feeling stressed or down. My advice to you is to realize it is ok to ask for help. No matter what you are struggling with, there is always someone to help. Whether it is family or friends, or a support group or counseling, don't try to combat stress all alone. Just the act of talking with someone will bring a fresh perspective and comfort to you. Many people feel they can handle everything on their own; they feel like a failure of sorts if they need to reach for help. I look at it from a completely different perspective. I applaud individuals who ask for help in order to better themselves and improve their lives. They see the long term gains. You have my permission to seek help this week if you need it.

Remember that no one is immune to stress. Life will always throw curve balls your way. For me personally, I rely heavily on my family and girlfriends. Getting a different perspective is essential in facing situations and being able to move past them. I value their opinions and respect what they have to say. Leaning on people is healthy as long as you don't depend on them to face challenges for you. You can seek advice, ask for support, and then you need to stand on your own two feet.

SIMPLIFIED HELP

*I don't want to bother anyone
I understand this concern. You may feel a twinge of guilt asking for help. Remember that people love to help each other, it makes them feel needed. So by reaching out to someone, you are in essence validating their opinions and assistance. You are making them feel special too. It is a win-win situation. There is a difference between asking for help all the time, and reaching out every now and then. If this is foreign to you, start small. When feeling stressed, ask for minor favors. Get comfortable with this before moving on to larger things. Taking it slow will help you feel more at ease as you go.

*I don't have time to eat healthy all the time
Let me preface this by saying you don't have to do anything one hundred percent of the time. If you make healthy choices eighty percent of the time, then the other twenty percent you can be a bit more relaxed. I also don't buy the excuse that you don't have time to make healthy choices. It is simply a matter of priority. Making healthy choices is just a lifestyle decision that may take a bit more preparation. Bulk up on healthy snacks and meals for the week and plan ahead. You should always have cut up vegetables and fresh fruit handy to grab as a snack. Have granola bars, cheese sticks, crackers, yogurt and other essentials at home. Bring lunches with you to work. Lack of preparation will lead you to grab something fast and convenient. And these choices are typically not very healthy. Take the time to embrace a healthy lifestyle and I guarantee you will have more energy to cope with everything life throws at you.

SIMPLIFIED AFFIRMATIONS

"I am completely capable of dealing with life's stressors"

"I have people in my life to support and help me when I need it"

"My body is healthy and capable of supporting me through any challenge"

"I am able to let go of stress and find the joys in my life"

   This week was important in order to give you the tools to face life's ups and downs. We all have choices as to how we respond to stress. Some people are good about rolling stress off their shoulders, while others carry it with them like the plague. I want you to realize the power each and every one of you has in coping with pressure. By using resources available to you, reaching out to others, and maintaining a healthy mind and body, you will be well-equipped to live a relatively stress free life. Good luck!

Week 9

Improve body language and boost your confidence

How many of you believe that your body language affects your confidence and the way you feel at any given moment? Think of the statement, *emotion is created by motion.* If you sit for a long period of time your natural energy levels automatically lower. And what happens when you get up, walk around a bit and return to your seat? You have more energy and you give yourself a boost. It is so important to move and be aware of your body language. I know firsthand the effects of standing tall and being active every day. I have always been on the tall side, and when I was younger I was a bit insecure about this trait. I would hunch over and try to make myself shorter. My mother would constantly remind me to stand tall and proud. Her constant reminders finally paid off, and I was able to stand tall, thus improving my posture, without thinking twice. I come across as someone confident and self assured. I also physically feel better from the movement. If I sit for too long of a period of time, I get grumpy and restless.

When you act confident, you send positive vibes to those around you. Even if you are not feeling extremely confident, act as though you are. So, how do you do this? Walk tall and with purpose. Gesture with your hands when you talk, and remember to smile. Smile as you walk down the street, when you talk to others, even when you are alone in front of the mirror. You will be surprised how much better you feel and it will project a positive image to all those around you. This image will attract opportunities and positive people your way. The way we communicate in our appearance, posture, gestures, gaze and expression can be such a powerful tool in the way we feel and react to others. Fake it until you feel it. If you do not feel confident, act is if you do. Over time you will carry the traits of someone extremely confident. What traits do people who are self assured have? They stand tall. They put effort into their appearance. They communicate well with others. They know what they want.

I worked with a client Tammy who was a bit on the insecure side. She came to her appointments in sweats and baseball caps, and she rarely smiled. She was a fascinating woman, but she was not playing to her strengths. She wondered why she was still single and working at a job that she disliked. She did not devote time to exercise, and she ate foods out of convenience. She had so many natural talents that she wasn't tapping into. I asked her to try an experiment with me. For one month I wanted her to act, breathe, and personify someone who was very confident and self assured. She listed for me characteristics of someone who was confident, and it was her job to become this person for the next four weeks. She was on for the challenge. The first thing she did was get rid of her current way of dressing. She needed to dress professionally, even if she was just going to the store. She then realized she was in desperate need for a haircut and makeover. These changes then led her to smile more. She realized confident people were generally happy and upbeat. She then began working out with a trainer. She saw confidence as having internal and external strength. Her next task was changing her behavior at work and communicating more with her superiors. She started offering more ideas and bringing more to the table. She also engaged in more dialogue with her colleagues. So, guess what happened to Tammy after one month of faking confidence? She realized she wasn't faking anymore. She felt confident. Her appearance improved, she was smiling more, and she even got promoted at work. Her superiors had no idea she was as creative and bright as she was, because she never let them see her in that way. Her entire life changed because of one experiment where faking something turned into her reality.

Remember that you, too, can boost your confidence by simply changing your body language. Too many people play the victim role if they are lacking self confidence. Initially, someone else made them feel the way they do, or they have always been insecure, so that is the way they assume it will always be. Do not be so quick to give your power away. Why not take control of how you feel and make the necessary changes to improve how you see yourself. You have nothing to lose by faking confidence this week. Why not give it a try and see how you feel. See if you would change things in your life to accommodate this confidence. Maybe you would dress differently. Possibly you would get a makeover. Perhaps you would make the time for exercise instead of sitting on the couch every evening. I want you to be aware of your body language this week and see if it needs some improving.

ACTION STEPS FOR THE WEEK

1. Dress to win

This week I want you to focus on your appearance. Ask yourself these questions: Do I feel confident? Do I look confident? What could I do with my appearance to give myself the edge? What areas of your appearance are you uncomfortable with? What are the pros and cons of not doing anything about it? I want you to be proactive when it comes to your appearance. Unfortunately someone's first impression is your outward appearance. They have nothing else to judge, because they do not know you yet. So, make the first impression a good one, and then they will have the opportunity to see the "real" you. The time and effort you invest will go leaps and bounds in your favor. Make a list of the things you would like to improve, and then pick one at a time. Get to work!

2. Smile, smile, smile

Smile a lot more than you have been doing. Just the art of smiling will change your mood and demeanor. When you are talking with people this week, look them straight in the eye. This will create an aura of confidence and assurance. When you are insecure and down, what is the last thing you feel like doing? Smiling? Why, of course. You don't feel happy, so why on earth would you fake a smile? Because faking a smile will lead you to feelings that promote more smiles. You can't help but feel better when you have a smile on your face. Smiling will make you come across as more approachable and confident. You have nothing to lose by experimenting this week. On the flip side, the more you frown, the worse you feel. By not smiling, you are giving in to insecurities and unhappiness. Something so basic and simple has the power to impact your life in a huge way.

3. Keep on moving

Focus on moving this week. Moving creates what? Yes, emotion. Be aware of your body language both at home and at work. Make an effort to move more, stand taller, and keep the energy flowing. The movement part is critical in body language and confidence. The more you slouch or sit, the fewer endorphins you have running through your body. These endorphins give you a natural high that promote self confidence. Instead of going straight to the television when you get home from work, go for a brisk walk. I guarantee you will feel better and more refreshed. Try to move a little bit every day. Take the stairs instead of the elevator. Go for a morning jog. Get some fresh air in the middle of a work day. Commit to moving on a daily basis. This week prioritize making time for movement, even if it is just ten minutes here and there. When you least feel like moving, tap into an inner strength to motivate yourself. Good luck!

This week was about discussing body language and confidence. There have been many times in my own life when I didn't realize the impact of my body language on myself or others around me. I didn't realize that slouching radiated a lack of confidence on my part. Sometimes just the act of being aware of your body language helps you make some necessary changes. If you slouch, or rarely smile at others, or radiate an energy that is not very welcoming, you may want to work on that this week.

SIMPLIFIED HELP

*I just don't believe changing my body language will boost my confidence

If you have severe confidence issues that have been with you for quite some time, you may need to tap into several resources. Seeking a therapist or counselor who specializes in your situation may be a great first step. However, changing your body language and bringing more activity into your life will definitely move you in the right direction.

Just like my client Tammy, if you fake confidence for a while and do what it takes to make yourself feel better, you absolutely will increase your morale. My belief is that doing *something* is better than *nothing*. Try acting the part, thus living a life like someone confident and self assured, and see if it rubs off.

* I feel certain habits are stuck with me

Let's say you are someone who rarely looks a stranger in the eye. When you encounter someone new, you look away or you look down at your feet. Just start with subtle changes and work your way up. Start by focusing on people you know. Try to maintain eye contact and look up when walking around. Once you are comfortable with this, use the same tactics with strangers. If you are in an elevator, smile at the person and look ahead. When walking down the street, look straight in front of you and acknowledge people who pass you by. See how much better you feel by incorporating these simple acts of positive body language.

SIMPLIFIED AFFIRMATIONS

"I am confident and self assured"

"I am confident in my abilities and what I have to offer the people around me"

"I am always working on improving myself and my self-assurance"

"I have the tools to boost my confidence from the inside out"

Please journal specific ways you can improve your body language and confidence.

1.

2.

3.

4.

5.

Remember it is ok to start small and work your way up. Making even subtle changes will give you the confidence to do more. Your body language is the attitude and energy you give off to others around you. By smiling more, standing taller and engaging more with people, you will see a shift in how others react to you. Their reactions will ultimately boost your confidence and open possibilities that were once closed off. Take back your power and do what it takes to feel comfortable in your own shoes.

Week 10

Just go for it!

How many of you have desperately tried to make changes in your life, only to get stuck before you even began? Maybe losing weight has been an ongoing battle for you. Possibly venturing out for a new career has been on your mind. Perhaps seeking Mr. or Mrs. right has been a constant desire for you. But, that is as far as it went. You have great desires, but the motivation or drive just isn't there. How many times did you recite the phrases "I'll start tomorrow," or "I'll start next Monday" in your head? I am guilty of this myself at times. Sometimes you are just clearly unmotivated to do anything, and if this is every now and then it would not be a big deal. However, if you tell yourself these phrases all the time, thus not doing anything, then it does become a big deal.

It is easy to come up with excuses to put off your dreams, goals and aspirations. Otherwise there would be no need for personal trainers, life coaches, therapists or self help guru's in the world. Where have these excuses gotten you? The exact same place you are today and the same place you will be tomorrow if you do not do something about them. Why not 'just go for it' for once and for all? Why not commit to taking action ***today***, not tomorrow, even if it's very small steps. Stop waiting for your life to change ***for*** you, ***you*** need to change your life. Something I am always reciting to my clients is that I do not want them to have regrets down the road. I do not want them to look back and wish they had done something that they clearly had the opportunity to do now. I do not want them to be at the same cross roads one year from now that they could have crossed through now.

A very attractive young woman in her mid-thirties came to me miserable in a relationship. She had been unhappy for years, but did not know what to do. She was with this man for ten years, unhappy for eight of them, but was afraid to move on. She was stuck in the comfort of being with someone, even if it was the wrong someone. So, I asked her if she would be ok if she was still unhappy and miserable one year from now. She of course said no, and this began our journey together. She finally gained the strength and confidence to move on into single hood, and when she did, she wondered why she didn't do it years ago. The saying 'just go for it' was something she couldn't do back then. She needed the support and advice to know she would be ok.

Sometimes it helps to look at what you can accomplish every day, instead of looking at the large picture. Looking at a goal in its entirety is sometimes so overwhelming that it stops you in your tracks. Let me give you a prime example from my own life. One of my best girlfriends convinced me to sign up for the MS150 bike ride. It is a hundred-fifty mile bike ride ridden over two days to raise money for MS. I love riding my bike, so I was excited for this. However, I was used to going on simple six to eight mile rides, not seventy-five mile rides. After training for a couple of months, and let me explain what a major challenge this was for me, the day of the race arrived. Knowing that I not only had to survive seventy-five miles of unknown territory, but I had to wake up the next morning and do it all over again, was a bit daunting. If all I focused on was the fact that I would be sitting on my bike nonstop for six to seven hours, I would not have even started the ride. Luckily, the organizers of the ride were brilliant. They had rest stops every ten miles or so, packed with snacks and bathrooms. This was my saving grace! All I had to focus on was getting to the next rest stop. My goal was broken down from seventy-five miles to ten-mile increments. I didn't even allow myself to consider how much further I had to go. All I focused on was getting to the next stop. Just so you know, I finished the race, all one-hundred-fifty miles of it. My body performed beautifully and I am proud that I pushed myself and stuck to it.

This example goes to show that anything is possible if you just break a goal down into bite-size chunks. Don't set yourself up to fail by creating unrealistic expectations. The "just go for it" mentality applies to doing **something**, rather than **nothing**. *A woman, Stacie, came to me* *with hopes of losing some weight and embracing a healthier lifestyle. She had always fought her weight and struggled with feeling unaccepted and unloved by others, especially her own family. She knew what she needed to do, but she always procrastinated getting things started. She was solely focusing on losing fifty pounds, and that thought terrified her. What would happen if she lost the weight? How would her life change? Would she then have to face her feelings that she's pushed aside for so long? After working together for a month or so, we set up a plan that she felt comfortable with. She started working out at her company gym and brought sack lunches instead of eating at the cafeteria. These simple changes motivated her to do more. She hired a personal trainer and also began setting boundaries with people in her life. Her life dramatically improved. This all happened because she was tired of the excuses. She realized she had the power to take small steps in the right direction.* This week I want you to instill the "just go for it" attitude as well. No more putting off what you can start today. If you knew your life was going to end soon, would you put things off? Of course not! You would do now what you wouldn't be able to do at a later date. So, live your life fully in the here and now. Do not wait for something to happen before you get fully engaged in your life.

ACTION STEPS FOR THE WEEK:

1. Where is the procrastination?

What specific areas of your life have you procrastinated on? Write in this space what you wish to improve. For example (losing weight, saving money, changing careers, leaving a bad relationship.)

_____

_____

_____

_____

_____

_____

_____

_____

_____

How are you benefiting by procrastinating? How would your life be different if you acted on this list? What are you so afraid of? Start to peel the layers away so you can get to the real reasons why you are stuck.

2. One year rule

If you have had a goal for over a year and still not progressed or achieved it, it might be time to let it go or reinvent it. Sometimes we fail to achieve goals because they are the wrong goals. If you are not excited or passionate about the goal at hand, the likelihood that you will achieve it diminishes. Let's say you have a goal of getting to the gym a couple times a week to exercise. For some reason you can't motivate yourself to go. Maybe the gym is just not the place for you. Maybe you prefer being outdoors. Forcing yourself to do something you clearly don't enjoy is not going to help. Instead, get involved in an outdoor activity, like biking or joining a walking or running club. Maybe you have always wanted to try rock climbing. There is no set way to get exercise into your life, do what you enjoy and you will reap the benefits.

3. Just go for it!

Commit this week to having the "just go for it" attitude. Instead of procrastinating, just do something that leads you in the right direction. When you find yourself excusing the inaction, stop and make the choice to go forward now not later. If you have a hard time with this, instill the help of some friends or family members. Having some accountability from someone other than yourself will give you the boost and support you need. When I was riding the MS150, going up mountain after grueling mountain, it would have been easy to give up. I did not however want to tell my children that I didn't finish the ride. They witnessed my training and were rooting for me the entire weekend. That kept me going. Do whatever it takes to create the support you need to succeed!

I know how feeling alone at times can turn to a fear of asking for help. Just remember that if a goal is important enough to you, you will find the means to make it happen. Going for it is about taking one step after another, not worrying about the destination, just surviving the journey. Just go at your own pace, because it is your life and your journey, no one else's. As long as you are at peace with the direction your life is taking, then so be it.

SIMPLIFIED HELP

* I don't have the strength to go for it

I do believe that timing is critical in life. If you feel that you are at a point in your life where you don't have the strength to move forward, please don't hesitate to ask for help. I know how it feels to hit rock bottom. I was at that very place after my mother died. It took all of my energy just to get out of bed every morning. Luckily I had a great support group of friends and family that got me through that time in my life. I knew there was absolutely no way I would survive on my own. Please know there are always resources and individuals prepared to help in any way they can. Reach out your hand when you cannot do it on your own.

*I have "gone for it" time and time again and it has not gotten me anywhere

Then it means you need to continue going for it, until you reach your desired goal. Some people in life make things look easy, and it very well may be easy for them. Don't compare! I guarantee you are stronger and more resilient by having the courage to keep going. Did you know that the definition of *crazy* is doing something over and over, yet expecting a different result? Maybe you need to go about things in a different manner. Spice it up a bit. Try something new. Don't expect that a goal will finally be achieved by trying over and over with the same approach. Be willing to look outside the box.

SIMPLIFIED AFFIRMATIONS

"Every day I have the strength to persevere"

"I am surrounded by individuals who support me to be my best"

"I am willing to look outside the box for answers yet to be seen"

"Every day I am moving closer to a purpose-driven life"

"I have the strength to conquer whatever comes my way"

This week is about tapping an inner strength that we are all born with. No one is more special or deserving of having a wonderful life; it is your gift of just being. It is the *action* that is missing in so many individuals equations. You want something so bad, the intentions are good, but the action steps are absent. You need to act on what you want. Create a plan and stick to it. Instill help from others in order to keep you on track. I support you fully to create the life and achieve the goals that would bring you happiness and fulfillment. You have the means to make it happen.

Week 11

Key to success

What do you think the key to success is? Is it money, prestige, skill, desire or attitude? Or is it a combination of all of the above? All of these have a bearing on success. However, your attitude does much to define your level of success. I am a believer that your attitude and the energy you exude is a direct correlation to your level of success in life. You may portray all of the items listed; however your attitude determines what you do with them. I truly believe you cannot succeed with a losing attitude. Even if you have monetary success, but you are negative and bitter, success has little value. I also believe you cannot fail with a winning attitude. If you are upbeat, optimistic and full of life, you are a success no matter how others define it. I have worked with individuals who on the outside appeared to be very successful. They had the lifestyle of wealth and elegance, but were miserable. I have also worked with people who had very simple lives, but were successful in their own right.

What creates your attitude? Your outlook on life creates your attitude. You can look at everything that occurs in your life as positive and meaningful, and strive to make the best of every situation. Or, you can view difficult times in your life as complicated and meaningless, and let yourself be defeated by them. The viewpoint is yours to choose. I also believe success is instilling a burning desire to accomplish certain life goals. This desire will help you overcome obstacles and roadblocks along the way. Having the right attitude and strong desire are essential elements of success.

I was blessed to grow up in a home filled with love and financial security. I saw first hand from my father what education and hard work could provide. I also learned from my mother the importance of following your passions and surrounding yourself by solid and loving friends. This foundation defined for me at a very young age what success looked like. Success for me was financial security, good friends and family, and living a passion and purpose-driven life. If my life were to consist of only one of the above, I would not feel complete and whole. It is important for each one of you to look at your own upbringing and define what success means to you. Witnessing my mother overcome illness after illness, with an absolutely admirable and positive attitude taught me the importance of attitude. Her attitude and positive outlook helped her overcome breast cancer twice and stage four ovarian cancer. Even through the most difficult and disheartening times, she held her head high. Please know that your attitude is one of very few things you have complete control over in your life. You choose what kind of attitude you want to embody.

Joe came to see me wanting clarity on why he was so unhappy. If you met Joe, you would assume he was extremely successful. He was attractive, smart, financially secure and healthy. After a couple of sessions together, it became abundantly clear to me why Joe was not satisfied. He was divorced after ten years of marriage to his college sweetheart. I asked Joe to define success to me. He explained that he admired his parents' marriage and when he was younger he vowed to create a similar marriage one day. Even though he had much success in business, without his life partner it did not mean much to him. Success to him meant having a loving family, plain and simple. And he had lost that element. After working together he found the tools that were buried inside him. He made some changes and reprioritized how he spent his time. He began dating and met a wonderful lady. He was determined to live the rest of his life in his parent's honor by spending more time on things that mattered most to him.

Know that there is no set definition of success. Success means something different to everyone, so create your own definition. Integrate a positive attitude and see where it leads you. You may be surprised by your desire to change course. If you feel successful, then do not worry about what others think. Too often we get so wrapped up in others opinions, we lose sight of what matters most. If your parents always wanted you to become a doctor, but you had a passion for teaching, follow your own heart. This is your life and your happiness, so try not to live it for others. Create a successful life based on decisions that you make on your own.

ACTION STEPS FOR THE WEEK

1. Define success

Take some time this week defining what success means to you. Is it defined by how much money you make? Is it personal achievement? Is it being acknowledged by peers? You need a clear definition before you can set out to create and achieve it. Even though my mother's life was cut far too short, I guarantee she would say she lived a very successful life. She had a loving family, she surrounded herself by great friends, she laughed a lot, she followed her passions, and she did not let fears dictate the course of her life. She attained more success in fifty years than most attain in a lifetime. I am so grateful for such a remarkable role model.

Success to me looks like

_____

_____

_____

_____

_____

_____

2. Look at your attitude

What role does your attitude play in your life? Are you a "cup is half full" or "cup is half empty" kind of person? Take a look at how your attitude affects your ability to cope in various situations. Everyone is dealt difficulties in life, some more than others, however, it is how you respond that sets you apart. I am sure you all know someone that is always optimistic. No matter what life throws at them, they keep a positive attitude and outlook. In the end they will always succeed in their own way. Your upbeat attitude is the glue that will always hold you together and instill faith when things get difficult. Because I am a positive person, I have been able to instill the same values and outlook in my children. Hopefully they will look back on their life with the same admiration and appreciation for the lifestyle and beliefs my husband and I gave them, that my parents gave me.

3. Make the changes

Now that you have taken the time to define success and recognize the role attitude plays in your life, it is time to act. Nothing will ever change unless you put action into the equation. Are you currently experiencing a successful life, as defined by your above statements? If not, what changes need to be made? Do you need to rearrange how you spend your time? Do you need to make some more drastic life changes? What about your attitude and outlook? Do you need some help seeing the blessings in difficult times? Make a list of changes you are willing to implement.

1.

2.

3.

4.

5.

6.

7.

8.

9.

10.

If my life ended today, I would have to say that I would have no regrets. I have lived a very successful life. I have an amazing family, good health, a job I love, and fantastic friends. By my own definition, I am a success. Make sure the life you live is one of your choosing. Define success and then take it upon yourself to create that life. The only thing stopping you is self-imposed hurdles or giving in to circumstances. I support you in creating your best life!

SIMPLIFIED HELP

*I was never raised with the confidence to succeed

I understand that your upbringing plays a huge role in your current beliefs and outlook on life. I have worked with many individuals who struggled with getting rid of past negative beliefs that played over and over in their heads. I have also witnessed the power of changing your beliefs into more positive and empowering thoughts. Even if you were not raised with the knowledge that you can succeed in anything you put your mind to, does not mean you can't break through those barriers and create a wildly successful life. Re-create your own belief system to one that supports your dreams. If you are having a hard time doing this on your own, instill some help. Work with a trained therapist or life coach. Join a support group. Talk with your good friends and family. Just don't give in to circumstance as the blueprint for the rest of your life. Now as adults, we have the power to make decisions that are in our best interest.

*My definition of success is distorted

Maybe you have come to the realization that your definition of success is not one you believe in. Possibly your upbringing taught you that success was all about money and prestige. Maybe you believed that success had everything to do with power and control. And now you appreciate the fact that success is something totally different. Letting go of those deep-rooted beliefs is hard to do. Maybe your social circle and family still believe success is all about superficial achievements and it is hard for you to walk away from this group. Remember you don't have to turn your back on all of these people; you just have to stand tall in your own beliefs. Make sure you live your life according to your own rules, not the rules someone instilled upon you.

SIMPLIFIED AFFIRMATIONS

"I am living a successful life on my own terms"

"People are coming into my life to help me create joy and happiness"

"I have the tools and support to create powerful and positive beliefs"

"I have the power to choose the path I take in life"

You have the opportunity now, today, to make changes in your life. No one can do this for you. People can love, support, and help you, but ultimately it is up to you. The fact that you picked up this book says that you have the desire and know-how to make some powerful changes. Go at your own pace and don't be afraid to face fears along the way. You will gain strength and momentum every time you do just that. Have a great week and congratulations on your progress so far.

Week 12

Live a life of no regrets

A wish I have for all my clients, colleagues and friends is that they live a life of no regrets. More specifically I am referring to the relationships in your life, both past and present. My mother has been gone for thirteen years, and one thing I know for sure is that I feel complete peace with our relationship. Through our ups and downs she always knew how much I loved and adored her, and vice versa. Particularly toward the end of her life, I never hesitated to express my feelings for her. She knew she was cherished above all else. I was in my early twenties when my mother was first diagnosed with Lou Gehrigs disease. It was not even a question in my mind that I would devote any amount of time and energy helping my mom in any way she needed. My life was put on hold for a couple of years, but I do not regret one moment of that time, for it was probably the most cherished and significant time in my life. Bringing comfort to my mother, such as sleeping next to her at night, helping her use the restroom, blending foods for her feeding tube, and getting beaten by her at Scrabble, became my daily schedule. I put my emotions aside to be her strength when she most needed it. And I will never have any regrets; quite the opposite. I am blessed that I had that time with her, and I know she was grateful that I was able to be there.

I am sharing these memories for the sole purpose of helping others live a life of no regrets. In some situations, you will not get a second chance. You do not know what tomorrow will bring, so make amends and express your feelings now while you have the opportunity. In some situations, there are hurt feelings involved. You can choose to hold your ground and wait for someone else to apologize first, or you can take the high road and make a difference here and now. No matter what the outcome, you will be better off for taking the first step. If I asked you right now to tell me what regrets you would have if your life ended tomorrow, what would you say? This pertains solely to people in your life. Would you regret not apologizing to a friend for something you did years ago? Would you have regrets about being unfaithful to someone you loved? Would you regret not sticking up for a friend who needed your support? Take a minute to write down what, if any, regrets come to mind.

I regret _____

_____

_____

_____

_____

I know that it is easier sometimes to let your pride get in the way. My husband will be the first to acknowledge that I sometimes have a hard time being the first to say "sorry." I have gotten much better over the years, but I have to manage my stubborn streak from kicking in. Never allow being stubborn to get in your way of being honest with your feelings.

I have talked with many people over the years who have regrets. They regret not being more present in their children's lives. They regret working so much. They regret losing touch with a friend. They regret not following their passions. There is only one positive outcome to admitting your regrets. Hopefully the regret opens your eyes to what really matters in your life, and it gives you the motivation and drive to change course. Do not wait until it is too late. That is the worst feeling. If you have the time to make amends now, do it. If you wait too long you may not have the opportunity, and then you will have the guilt as well to deal with.

Jeffrey came to see me when he hit a low point in his life. He always struggled with his relationship with his father. He never felt validated or loved unconditionally. Because of this, he drifted from his dad and moved on with his life. He eventually got married and had children, and this transition motivated him to make amends for the sake of his family. He wanted his children to have the opportunity to create their own relationship with their grandfather, despite his feelings. He kept putting off the phone call telling himself he would do it the following week. Well the following week never came. His father had a massive stroke and passed away before he had the chance to speak with him. Jeffrey could not forgive himself and was in a serious funk when I met with him. He felt such sadness, not necessarily for himself, but for his children. He knew he waited too long and this was something he had to live with for the rest of his life. We worked together on forgiveness and bringing closure to the situation. After quite some time Jeffrey was able to feel peace. He learned more about his father from his mother. He got out photo albums and allowed his children to get to know their grandfather in their own way. This is clearly one of those times that he wished he could go back in time. This week I want you to review your own life and determine if there are any personal regrets that you can amend.

ACTION STEPS FOR THE WEEK:

1. Make amends

I want you to start with yourself first. Forgive yourself for things in your past that you have held on to. It's time to let it go. To err is human. We all make mistakes and it would be naïve to think otherwise. Sometimes we are too hard on ourselves and we expect more than we should. Most of us did the best we could with the tools we were given. Of course we learn and mature as we grow older. Have you held on to guilt for something far too long? I want you to list what areas or experiences need your forgiveness.

I am willing to forgive myself for

_____

_____

_____

_____

_____

_____

You need to be willing to forgive yourself first before forgiving others. This is also an opportunity to forgive your own mistakes before making amends with others you may have hurt.

2. Look at your past

Who in your past do you still hold grudges against? Who do you have unresolved issues with? If your life ended tomorrow, who would you regret not talking to? I want you to write down the names of everyone who is still an emotional drain. Make a commitment to create peace instead of toxicity. Holding on to past hurts and pains keeps you in the past; you are never fully free to move forward in your life. You have two choices here. You either accept what happened, and peacefully let it go. Or, make things right by apologizing and opening lines of communication to resolve what happened. Do not stand in the middle and hope things will get better on their own. Who do you need to make amends with? List their names below.

*
*
*
*
*
*
*

This week decide what course of action you feel comfortable pursuing.

3. Say you're sorry and forgive

Now is your opportunity to bring peace and closure to the relationship. Either take the high road and apologize-even if you were not in the wrong, or forgive them for their wrong doing. You will release a tremendous weight off your shoulders and feel much better. You can either choose the emotional drain of carrying these negative feelings with you, or you can choose to let it go and move on. What can you do to feel better about making the first move? I want you to accept that the outcome of this conversation is not the intention; you have no control over how the other person will respond. You will however, stand taller and more fulfilled just by being mature enough to make the first move.

As a teenage girl, I, of course, completely acted as if the world was going to come to an end if a girlfriend or boy did something to hurt me. I would act so stubborn and unforgiving and my mother frequently tried to help me see things from a different angle. She would constantly point out that I needed to put my pride aside to move on. My pride, she said, would just keep me in a place of anger and hurt. What are you gaining by holding on to past anger? Would making amends allow you to move on with your life? Would you be healthier emotionally and physically? It is up to you, but my advice is to try forgiveness and see how you feel.

SIMPLIFIED HELP

* My hurt far outweighs my ability to make amends

I can understand how deep rooted some hurts can feel. I also understand how difficult it can be to move on sometimes. You simply may not be in a place right now where you can forgive and move on. Maybe you are too close to the experience to move on. If something happened recently, you may need some time to process everything and grieve in your own way first. If plenty of time has passed, however, it may be time to let it go. By making amends, you are not approving the behavior, you are just allowing yourself the freedom to move on. The hurt, pain and anger keep you stuck. See what steps you can take this week to move forward into a place of peace and understanding.

*I have no desire to make amends with this person

Like I mentioned before, there is no rule that you have to make amends with anyone. If you genuinely have no desire to reconcile or make peace, that is completely your decision. As long as you are at peace with that decision and you are able to live your life fully in the present, then that is ok. As long as you know you won't regret a decision later in life, then you are not being dragged down emotionally. Just take some time this week to reflect on your past and your feelings, and then decide if anything needs to be done.

SIMPLIFIED AFFIRMATIONS

"I am at peace with everyone in my life"

"I am living a life of no regrets"

"I have released past anger and resentment; it no longer consumes me"

"I forgive myself for any past wrong doings; I did the best I could at the time"

"I am continuously working toward forgiving others"

I work with many individuals who are consumed with regrets from their past, particularly with other people. They stayed in a relationship too long. They didn't stand up for themselves in a friendship. They never reconciled with a loved one. Life is very short and sacred. I want you to feel ok with your decisions and behaviors in life. When you approach your later years, you don't want to be consumed with regret and remorse. I want you to look back and feel great about the life you led and the people you surrounded yourself with. Please take some time this week to mull over whether or not you need to make amends with anyone from your present or past. I wish you luck with this homework. I know each and every one of you can make huge strides if the desire is great enough.

Week 13

$\mathcal{M}$ake a life list

If you knew with complete certainty that you were going to take your last breath tomorrow, what would you do? Would you call all of your loved ones? Would you travel the globe? Would you spend some time thinking about everything you wish you had done in your life? We all have dreams and visions of what we will do "someday." But when is "someday?" The fact is that most of us have no idea exactly what tomorrow will bring. The past is in the past and so the only guarantee is the here and now. Why not take the time to list everything that you've always dreamed of accomplishing in your life. Randy Pausch, who became famous after his "Last Lecture," knew with certainty that his life was coming to an end. He lived his life more fully in his forty seven years, than most of us live in several lifetimes. He made his life list and actively engaged in achieving the majority of the items on his list. He didn't have "someday" like the majority of us do.

I do not want this list to be a list of "shoulds," such as *I should lose weight*, or *I should give up smoking*, or *I should exercise more*. This is your ***think big*** list of activities or dreams that have taken a back burner in your life. Have you dreamed of scaling a fourteener for as long as you can remember? Have you always dreamed of sailing around the Meditteranean Sea? When are you going to stop dreaming about it and start acting on it? Many individuals create these life lists and then put them away or forget about them all together. How amazing would it feel to actually commit to these dreams and make them a reality? How rewarding would it be? How would your life be different as a result of crossing these activities off your list? If most of us knew our time was coming to an end, I could almost guarantee that we would live more fully. We would pursue dreams now as best we could.

I have one client in particular who was flat out bored with her life. She was typically very active and ready for any challenge that was presented to her but she was in a rut. She loved the outdoors and thrived on pushing herself physically. I had her create her dream list of anything and everything she would love to achieve in her lifetime. I did not want her to filter this list in any way, it was her opportunity to dream big. She came up with twenty five items on this list, ranging from sky diving to climbing one fourteener every year to swimming with the dolphins. It was a great list! The next step was actively pursuing several of these activities. She picked a couple that were at the top of her list and starting creating specific goals to achieve them. She felt an excitement that she had not felt in years. Knowing that she was actually going to cross some of these items off her list was exhilirating. Once she got started, there was no slowing her down. She felt alive again and rejuvenated.

This week is about creating your own life list, a list of things you would love to achieve in your lifetime. Have fun with this list, don't hold yourself back. This is your opportunity to dream big and have fun. Something on my mother's wish list was swimming with the dolphins. Unfortunately she never got the opportunity due to her illnesses, but this is a dream I have incorporated on my own wish list. Someday I will swim with the dolphins and my mother will be there right along side me.

ACTION STEPS FOR THE WEEK:

1. Make your list

Throw away all of your old lists. Create a new life list of all the things you intend to achieve in this lifetime. I want you to have fun with this list and dream big. *You* are the biggest obstacle when it comes to making your dreams a reality. We have a tendency to self sabotage our dreams. You are responsible for creating and living out your dreams. Right now I want you to write down what first comes to your mind. You can expand on this list later.

I would love to achieve the following in my lifetime:

_____

_____

_____

_____

_____

_____

_____

_____

_____

_____

2. Break it down

Looking at your list and knowing where you are in your life right now, I want you to highlight the items that you can realistically achieve this year. The next step is to create a month by month blueprint on accomplishing these dreams. How can you break your dreams into smaller tasks? What would you need to do monthly or even weekly? Breaking down your goals will dramatically decrease your stress level and uncertainty of achieving them. Start by writing down the date you would like to achieve your goal by, and then work your way backwards to the current date.

3. Bring on support

It is critical to surround yourself by people and resources who will help you stick to your goals. When I trained for the MS150 bike ride, having my friends ride with me and push me was so important. I never could have succeeded without their constant support and encouragement. You need to tap into your resources and support structure. Possibly you need to join a support group or branch out. Do you have friends or colleagues with similar goals? That way you can hold each other accountable and it will be more gratifying. Try to brainstorm ways you can support yourself to succeed this time around.

Billy always wanted children. He knew he would be an extraordinary father and this goal unwavered over time. This was at the top of his wish list, however he still has not met a woman to settle down with. He always assumed he would get married and have children. He recognized that he could not wait for this to happen, so he needed to explore other options to realize his dream of having a child. He filled out papers to adopt and is currently waiting for a match. He may not have children in the customary fashion, but he is not willing to let this dream go. I am so proud of him and his ability to fulfill his dreams on his own terms.

SIMPLIFIED HELP

*I have never dreamed big and I do not know where to begin

I realize this week's assignment may be a bit out of your comfort zone, but it does not mean you can't try your best. If you have never dreamed big before, talk with friends and family about their own wish lists. You may get some wonderful ideas that you can take on as your own. Review your past and jot down ideas from things that brought you a lot of joy. What did you dream of as a child? What do people do now that bring up feelings of envy? You can start small and work your way up as you expand your ideas. Possibly it means you start by creating one dream and then go with that. See where that dream takes you.

*I don't have the financial means to follow my dreams

There are always creative ways to achieve goals. Maybe you can't achieve your dream next week, but who is to say you can't save money and create resources over the next year? Possibly it means volunteering in an organization that will give you opportunities. Maybe it is bringing on friends to help achieve the goal as a group. If you want something badly enough, you will find ways to make it happen. Perhaps it means taking your goal down a notch first. If my goal were to swim with the dolphins, maybe I would learn to scuba dive first or see if Habitat for Humanity needs volunteers in warm climates near the ocean. Tap into your creativity to see how you can move closer to your dreams.

SIMPLIFIED AFFIRMATIONS

"I am surrounded by people who are supporting my dreams and goals"

"I have the financial means to live and experience all of my wishes"

"People are coming into my life to help me follow my dreams"

"I am constantly following through on my life goals"

So what have you realized this week? Do you have a new appreciation for living your life to the fullest? Are you ready to embark on some of your life goals? Are you inspired to get to work? I want you to renew your passions and get engaged in the game of life. So many of us are so focused on the destination, that we completely miss the journey along the way. It is this journey that makes up our life, not the destination. My father is a constant reminder of living life to its fullest. He is always learning something new and living his life full of zest and purpose. He is such an inspiration that age is just a number. He lives more fully and with more joy than people half his age. I aspire to have his same outlook on life. Have a wonderful week and get to work!

Week 14

$\mathcal{N}$ow is the time to clean up your relationships

How does it feel to be surrounded by people who make you feel good about yourself? These people celebrate the person you are and support you to be the best you can be. On the other hand, how does it feel to be around people who drain your energy? These individuals focus on the negatives and provide very little encouragement or joy to the relationship. You have many choices in your life, but choosing who to surround yourself by is essential to your physical and emotional well-being. I have always been a fairly good judge of character and I can tell fairly quickly whether or not I want to pursue a relationship with someone. Life is just far too short to surround yourself by people who zap your energy. I have a great group of girlfriends and I value how we are able to fully support each other in our individual ventures.

I once worked with a lovely woman in her late thirties who knew she needed to make some drastic changes in her life. She was hanging out with women that were emotionally draining and negative. They had a tendency to gossip and put others down and my client was ready to move on. She didn't feel good when she was with them, but she didn't know how to severe the relationships. We worked on creating boundaries and boosting her self esteem so that she felt worthy of loving relationships. Doing the work gave her the confidence to make some changes. She slowly stopped investing time in the friendships and she focused on meeting new people. She felt a huge relief of pent up fear and she was finally able to create healthy and enriching relationships.

It is important to be honest with yourself whether someone in your life is contributing to or contaminating the relationship. Now is the time for you to re-evaluate the relationships in your life and determine a course of action. I want you to give yourself permission to spring clean the people in your life. You have the choice and ability to surround yourself by individuals who genuinely contribute to your growth and happiness. Just as you would spring clean the unnecessary items in your home every now and then, you can also spring clean relationships. People grow in different directions and sometimes choose to take separate paths. Sometimes we stay in relationships out of guilt or because it is easier that way. That is ok if that is your choice. However, if you know that it is in your best interest to break off the relationship, get the support you need to do just that.

Sometimes you may feel that a relationship is worth salvaging, and that you are not quite ready to let it go. If this is the case, then it is important that you set some clearer boundaries and let the other person know what changes need to be made. I was very good friends with a woman from college but our relationship was straining. Every time we talked she would be very pessimistic and down on herself. It got to the point that I didn't want to answer the phone or set aside time to get together. I did however treasure her as a person and I was willing to give her another chance if she made some changes. We met for lunch and I was honest with her about how our conversations always seemed down and depressing and I was at a point in my life where I needed to surround myself by positive and upbeat individuals. She was upset and a bit shocked and we parted ways. We didn't speak for a couple of weeks and then she gave me a call. She appreciated my honesty and said she would be conscious of the energy she gave off when she was with friends. She made a hundred-eighty-degree turn around and we are still good friends to this day. She was able to really look at herself and make some changes that deeply improved all of her relationships. This week I want you to look at the people in your own life and determine if a spring cleaning is in order. If you only surround yourself by loving and supportive people, then this may be a week you are able to easily move through.

ACTION STEPS FOR THE WEEK:

1. Make a list

Make a list of people who drain you physically and emotionally. This list should encompass people that take a lot from you, both time and energy. Sometimes these individuals are good at *taking* but not *giving* much in return. This list can involve people from work, friends, acquaintances, family members and lovers. I call these people "toxic" individuals, because they have a way of contaminating you spiritually and mentally. They do not offer much in a way of enriching your life. Don't feel bad if this is a long list, it just means you need to make some changes. In the space below, right the names that come to mind.

2. Decide which relationships are beneficial

Looking at your list, decide which relationships are worth saving. You may see potential with these people and so you are not willing to throw in the towel just yet. You may have feelings for these individuals and are willing to put forth the work to make it work. On the other hand, who are you willing to let go? There are probably some individuals from whom you have simply grown apart. Maybe you used to gossip a lot at work and now you don't feel the need to behave that way anymore. It might mean you part ways with the colleagues that act in this way, because you no longer get anything out of the relationships. Highlight the names above that you want to salvage.

3. Be true to yourself

The people you choose to surround yourself with are a true reflection of who you are and what you value in life. Choose wisely! I don't want you to settle for less than you deserve. Everyone deserves to be surrounded by people that respect them and want the best for them. If you want to save a relationship, it is important to have an open and honest conversation with the person. Express to them your desire to improve the relationship and then instill some boundaries for what *is* and *is not* acceptable anymore. If, on the other hand, you need to break off a relationship, it is also time to be honest. Communicate why it might be in everyone's best interest to part ways, and then stand tall and with purpose and class. It is nobody's fault, it is just time to move on.

Life is far too short to spend time and energy on things that don't have much value. If someone is negative, pessimistic, or self absorbed, it's not a good match for me. I cherish my friends and family, because they are a direct reflection of all that matters to me. We have very similar beliefs and values on what is most important in life, so we all feed off each others energy and insight. Seeing my mother fight for her simple joys through all of her illnesses, taught me the importance of not wasting any time. This includes relationships. If someone is holding you back from being the amazing being that you are, it's ok to stand tall and move on.

SIMPLIFIED HELP

*What if I am afraid of being alone, so I cannot leave a relationship?

Aren't you "alone" in a relationship that is not satisfying or rewarding? It is how you define alone. I would rather be alone and happy, than in a relationship that drains me physically and emotionally. Of course you may feel tremendous fear and trepidation at first, but it is all an opportunity for growth and spiritual advancement. Sometimes breaking through fears is the first step in creating a new life. You are allowing yourself the opportunity to walk through new doors and experience fresh things. Create a support group of people to help you through this. Lean on others to give you the strength when you may not have it.

*I can't leave all my friends, I'd have to start all over

Let me remind you that nothing worth anything ever comes easy. Is the end result worth the initial pain and uncertainty? If your entire group of friends is toxic and unhealthy, then you may have to make the difficult choice of starting completely fresh. We all need opportunities of rebirth in our lives, and this may be one of those. As difficult as it may be, you will come out a much more empowered and positive person. When you close one door, another door will present itself to you. Just remember that your "support team," the people you surround yourself by, is significant in your overrall happiness in life. Do what feels right to you.

SIMPLIFIED AFFIRMATIONS

"I am always surrounded by positive and loving people"

"I choose to create friendships with people that support my highest good"

"I am strong and resilient at all times"

"I am letting go of relationships that are not in my best interest"

"I always attract positive, loving, and supportive people into my life"

Julia came to see me about the time she was struggling with the decision to stay in a relationship or get out. She loved her boyfriend and had been with him for many years, but there was a deep sadness and disconnect between the two of them. They lacked the ability to have fun and she was a thrill seeker in every way. She knew deep down that he was holding her back from living the life she dreamed of. She just needed the support to leave her comfort zone and look more closely at what she needed in a relationship. After trying to make things better with her boyfriend, the nagging feeling didn't go away. She knew she needed to explore things on her own and find herself again. Months later she was completely engaged in life again, going on hikes and enjoying the outdoors. She was meeting new friends and feeling more confident every day. She knew it was time to let the relationship go, and once she gave herself permission to do so, she felt a huge relief in many ways.

Find your own inner strength this week and take the necessary steps to surround yourself by people who support you to be your best.

Week 15

Omit the negative voice in your head

Going through a typical day what does the predominant voice in your head sound like? Do you hear mostly encouraging positive words like "good job" or "you can do that?" Or are they self-defeating and negative such as "I can't believe you did that" and "you are not smart enough?" Sometimes we hear these words so often that we become immune to their impact on our daily lives and well-being. It is truly amazing how profoundly these words can affect all of the decisions we make in our life. Are you mainly guided by negative thoughts or supportive and loving thoughts? The first step is to become aware of the dialogue that goes on inside your head, and then you can choose to replace the negative dialogue with more constructive words.

When I was a sophmore in college I had a rough year. I didn't get into the sorority of my choice which at that age was a colossal blow to my confidence. I also got into several major car accidents which profoundly affected me. I was ok physically, but the emotional scars took a while to heal. Because of all this I gained a significant amount of weight, and this of course made me feel exponentially worse about myself. The dialogue in my head was less than loving and supportive, to say the least. When I went home for the summer, I decided enough was enough. I took it upon myself to regain my self worth again. I lost thirty pounds and felt great. I vowed never to lose myself like that again, and to this day I have kept my promise. I became more loving to myself and I realized at a young age how important it was to nurture my mind, body and spirit.

It is sad that we can be so hypercritical of ourselves, when we wouldn't dream of being that critical with a friend or family member. Why is that? Why do we hold ourselves to a lower standard? That voice in your head will critique your physical appearance, your personality, your social skills and so much more. On the flip side, how would it feel if you were your own biggest cheerleader? Wouldn't it feel empowering to rely on yourself to lift your spirits? You are simply breaking down the core of who you are when you constantly put yourself down. There are many things in life that you have absolutely no control over, such as natural disasters or dealing with ignorant people. The voice in your head however is completely under your control. You can pick and choose the words that fly around on a daily basis. Over time I guarantee you can release the harmful dialogue and bring on board more loving internal comments. It is all a matter of making the commitment to yourself to be more aware and constructive.

I asked a client Deliah to write down the dialogue that goes on in her head on a daily basis. Some of the comments consisted of "you are fat and ugly", "I can't believe how stupid you are", "you will always be a loner", and "you are so pathetic." These were just a handful of what she came up with. When we sat down and read all of her statements, she just cried. She couldn't believe how abusive she was to herself. She knew she was negative, but she had no idea to what extent. I explained that she could not expect others to treat her with kindness and respect until she was able to do that to herself first. She needed to respect herself enough so that she felt worthy of being treated kindly. She needed to do a complete overhaul of her inner voice. She was amazed how something so basic completely changed her in other ways as well. Once she started talking to herself with a more supportive tone, she decided to take it to the next level. She began nurturing herself physically and spiritually. She began exercising regularly, she fed her body healthier foods, and she got back on track with meditation. She felt better in so many ways and began attracting people into her life that treated her the same way.

It all starts with your mind and your thoughts, and then naturally other areas of your life are able to shift positively. Even if you were brought up in an unloving and unsupportive environment, you can still create new dialogue in your head. You can absolutely create new beliefs. I've seen it time and time again. I do not want you to give in to the fact that just because someone else told you you were unworthy or unattractive, that you need to believe those statements. Don't play that role for the rest of your life, create new beliefs and experiences. I support you fully in leaving certain beliefs in the past and establishing new ones for yourself. It is a matter of surrounding yourself by the right people, people who will support you in this new venture. This week I want you to become aware of the dialogue in your head, whether positive or negative. You will have the opportunity to decide whether or not something needs to be changed for the better.

ACTION STEPS FOR THE WEEK

1. Track your thoughts

I want you to keep a pad of paper with you for a couple of days and keep a record of how many times your negative voice goes off in your head. This includes criticizing yourself. Everytime you put yourself down, write a tally mark. Remember that you are only doing this exercise for a couple of days, so try not to think of it as a large task. Tracking your thoughts will give you a glimpse into your typical outlook on life. This exercise will determine whether you have many tally marks or just a couple here and there. Try to be as aware as you can, for this exercise is extremely helpful in making positive life changes. I've worked with many clients who had no idea they were so critical of themselves. This exercise was the first step in reprogramming their dialogue.

2. Replace these thoughts

Now that you are hopefully more aware of the negative expression in your head, it is time to replace these thoughts. I am a firm believer that likes attract likes, so the more you focus on the negative, the more you are attracting that energy into your life. I want you to create some positive affirmations that you say every time a negative thought pops into your head. The more often you state the positives, the more natural it will feel. Eventually you won't even have to think about it, you will just naturally say the positive statements to yourself. I want you to purchase some index cards. On the front of each card I want you to write a comment that goes through your mind on a regular basis. Maybe on one card you are going to write *"I am ugly and unattractive."* On another card you are going to write *"I will always be in debt."* Keep writing until you've gotten every negative statement written down. Now I want you to turn each card over and write the exact opposite of what you wrote. On the card where you wrote *"I will always be in debt,"* on the opposite side you will write something like *"I am always financially abundant."* So, you should eventually have a stack of cards with positive and affirming statements written on them. I want you to read these positive statements several times a day. Every time a negative statement goes through your mind, replace it with the positive one you came up with.

3. Be aware

This week I simply want you to be more aware. I want you to be more responsible with how you treat yourself and try to soften your tone. Just the act of being more aware will shift the way you see and talk to yourself. When you find yourself criticizing something, take a step back and change your dialogue. It is amazing what a difference being more "present" and aware can make in your life. Maybe you need visual reminders. Place sticky notes all over as a reminder to be kind to yourself. Place them on your bathroom mirror, or your refrigerator, your computer and your car. They will act as a cue to think positively.

Most people are much more critical of themselves than anybody else. For some reason we hold ourselves to such a lower standard. I work with mothers all the time who think they are doing a horrible job as moms . They feel like they have to be supermoms and do everything for everyone. *One client in particular had three children and ran a very busy household and business. She was constantly second guessing herself and yelling at her children. She therefore did not have a very nice dialogue going on in her head. She would put herself down incessantly and make herself feel even worse. Once we made some changes to her life that incorporated simplifying things and getting back on track with what really mattered, she was able to then focus on her inner voice. She realized she was doing the best she could, and she cut herself some slack. She began to nurture herself and this radiated to all those around her. Her life dramatically improved and she was able to get rid of the negative and disempowering voice in her head.* Now it is your turn to dissect how critical you are and take the necessary steps to sprinkle a little kindness fairy dust on yourself.

SIMPLIFIED HELP

* I have always been critical of myself and I do not know how to move past it

Remember that your upbringing plays a crucial role in how you act and behave today. If others showered you with insults and criticism's, then you are more likely to continue the cycle. However, you have the ability to break the cycle and create your own dialogue. If you are having a difficult time moving past the criticism's of yourself, reach out for help. There is absolutely nothing wrong with enlisting help when you need it. Seek out a therapist, life coach, clergy member, or counselor. This individual will help you release harmful dialogue while creating new discussions for that inner voice.

* I can say the positive words to myself, but I don't believe them

Like anything worth the wait, it is going to take a while before you truly begin to believe what you are saying. I don't want you to give up too early, that would be giving in before truly giving yourself a chance. If you had thirty years of self defeating dialogue, then of course it is going to take some time to turn that around. Don't expect a magic pill because it simply won't work in the long run. I want you to commit to stating positive affirmations to yourself until you begin to believe them. It may take a month, two months, or longer. I guarantee it will be well worth the effort.

SIMPLIFIED AFFIRMATIONS

"I am beautiful and perfect just the way I am"

"I am completely loved and accepted always"

"I am doing the best I can with what I am given"

"I accept myself for the person I am and the person I am becoming"

"I will always nurture and love myself unconditionally"

"I am always surrounded by people that love me and support me to be my best"

I want you to write down some specific affirmations that apply directly to you: Please read these daily~

_____

_____

_____

_____

_____

_____

_____

_____

_____

_____

I was blessed to be brought up in a loving home with two parents who cherished me and my siblings completely and individually. I have a sister and brother that are extremely bright and insightful. I always had to work a little bit harder for everything I got. It would have been easy to feel insecure and self-doubting in that atmosphere. My parents didn't allow this and they made sure that we each were loved completely for the strengths and gifts that we brought to the world. Therefore I never had time to doubt myself. I carried this self confidence and attitude of being able to achieve anything with me into adulthood. I realize that many people did not have a similar upbringing and so they struggle to leave the past in the past. The good news is that it is absolutely possible to create new self confidence and release inhibiting thoughts and behaviors. This week start the process of releasing the restrictive thoughts to make room for the encouraging ones.

Week 16

Passion is the key to a great life

It is easy to get caught up in the daily routine of tasks, responsibilities and chores, so that we forget to enjoy life's simple pleasures. The secret is creating a balance that provides for both sides of the equation. If you are able to embrace passion in your life, you are able to handle the rest with more ease. Whether you are passionate about the professional work you do, or the life you are living, you simply need passion in some form. My mother used the word passion a lot in her lifetime. She was not content with living an ordinary existence, she needed to enjoy things fully. She had many passions, some of which were getting her hands dirty in her garden and immersing herself in self-improvement. She loved going to workshops, talking with a wide variety of therapists or medical intuitives, or simply attending week-end seminars. She loved the experience of evolving as a person. She knew what her passions were and she naturally gravitated toward them. No matter how busy her life was, and I guarantee she seldom had a slow moment, she made the time to follow her passions.

Having something specifically for you, something that feeds your soul, is so important in creating an enriching life. Do you feel you are living a life immersing yourself in your passions? If your work is not your passion, are you able to fulfill it in other ways? So many people have a tendency to take care of other's needs first, but it is vitally important to take care of your own needs first. If you put your own desires and joys last, eventually you will have nothing left to give. Do you know why you are instructed to put your air mask on first in the event of an emergency on a plane? If you put an air mask on your child first and then something happens, you will be of no use to your children. You need to put the air mask on first, and then you are fully capable of helping your kids. This directly applies to pursuing your passions, so that you are complete and content, both emotionally and physically. When you are happy, those around you are happy. Finding the joy in life not only makes you a better person, but the positive energy you feel radiates to all those around you. I want you to be able to teach by example how important it is to pursue passion and joy in your life.

One of my clients, Caleigh, was struggling with providing for her children, working part-time, taking care of the home and many more tasks, so that she neglected her own needs in the process. She loved being a mother, but over the years she slowly lost part of herself along the way. She got so accustomed to giving to everyone else, volunteering at school, hosting parties, preparing family meals, and so forth, that she forgot what interested her. I asked her to compile a list of everything in life that she was passionate about, and she struggled with the exercise. She was embarassed to admit that she had no idea what her hobby's were. She had disengaged from them for so long, that she had to dig a little deeper to remember what brought her joy. By reviewing her past we were able to come up with some wonderful activities. The hard part was convincing her that commiting time to these activities was critical to her mental and emotional well-being. After working together for a couple of months, she saw first hand the benefits of getting engaged again in activities that she enjoyed. She felt a surge of joy and excitement that she had not felt for sometime. She had much more energy to give to her family and friends, and she was able to release the guilt of spending this time on herself.

I am a believer that living life without passion is just going through the motions of life without much feeling. Passion brings about purpose and meaning to everything you do. If I just went through my days engaging in activities that did not mean much to me, I would feel empty and incomplete. Over time this feeling would add up to sadness, depression, void, and insecurity. I have worked with many clients who did not prioritize passion-driven activities into their lives, and they felt sadness and lost. By following your organic passions, you will be guided in the right direction by the universe. I believe that things will click, you will meet the right people, and circumstances and opportunities will present themselves to you. This week I want you to get back in the game of life and bring your passions back.

ACTION STEPS FOR THE WEEK:

1. Plan for rediscovery

Make an effort this week to rediscover your innate passions. Listen to your inner voice. This voice will sometimes whisper to you a reminder of what is important and what makes you happiest in life. Maybe you are happy when you are outdoors and being active. Possibly you love to cook and entertain. Perhaps you love tapping into your creative side. I want you to keep a journal and write down everything that comes to mind that brings you peace and enjoyment. If you have a difficult time, I want you to review your past. What past time activities brought you a lot of joy? What did you do when you were younger that would make the time fly by? Take some time by yourself to really quiet your mind and see what comes up.

2. Take baby steps

Don't feel overwhelmed this week by trying to force your passions into your already hectic life. Take baby steps! Highlight a couple items off your list and commit to pursuing them at a pace that feels comfortable. You need to be willing to see the bigger picture and accept how these activities will benefit your life as a whole. Sometimes you need to simplify your life first before you plug in more activities. Take a look at your schedule and determine if there are activities that you can let go of completely or delegate to someone else. Making time for what really matters will be well worth the adjustment. These changes will ultimately create a life filled with purpose and balance. List the activities that you would like to pursue:

_____

_____

_____

_____

_____

_____

The best way to assure yourself that you will follow through with this task is to bring on some accountability. Ask a friend, colleague, or family member to check in with you on a regular basis. Accountability is huge when staying committed to a task or goal.

3. Go on a discovery mission

If you are having a hard time remembering what excites you, go on a discovery mission in your own home. The things we hold onto provide clues to our passions and genuine interests. What do you see that ignites these interests? Look at your bookshelf or DVD collection. Do you have a pile of photos and scrapbooks that you used to love putting together? Are there rollerblades in your garage that you used to love riding? Your home is a blueprint for what brings you joy, you just need to dig a little deeper. Take out a pad of paper and go explore your house. Write down whatever comes to mind, big or small. Do not think anything is petty. I don't want you filtering this list. You will be amazed what comes to the surface when you take your blinders off. Have fun!

My mother had a passion for bringing out the kid in her. She didn't believe being an adult meant putting all the fun and carefree activities aside. When she was in her early forties, she invited her close girlfriends over for a slumber party. They put on their pajamas, ate junk food, gave each other pedicures, and gossiped into the night. They had a blast! At the time I am sure I gave her a hard time, but looking back I admire her so much. She didn't live her life confined in a box, caring what others thought. She tapped into her passion and lived life fully. I hope to continue this pajama party tradition in her honor, and I am sure my kids will also think I am crazy and silly. Oh well, life is too short to concern yourself with what other people may or may not think. Enjoy your life in your own way.

SIMPLIFIED HELP

*I cannot push aside responsibilites to follow my passions

I am not asking you to relinquish all of your responsibilites and solely go after your dreams. I am asking you to create a balanced life, one that includes passion and purpose. You need to be responsible and take care of tasks, but it is also your responsibility to be happy, following what brings you joy. Life is not one or the other. There is a lot of gray matter in between. I have a lot of responsibilities as a wife, mother, daughter, sister and friend. But I also know how important it is to follow my own dreams and be true to myself. When my life is all over, following my dreams is a very important legacy I would like to leave. I would love everyone that I meet to remember me as a woman who lived a life of passion, purpose, vision, and lighthearted fun. So my wish for you is to release the guilt associated with following your passions. Create a life that has an equal balance of responsibility and genuine passion.

*I try to pursue my passions, but nothing satisfies me

Sometimes we throw in the towel a little too early. I've met and worked with many people that tried to pursue their interests, but they gave up before really seeing where it would take them. If you are continuously pursuing passions, but nothing seems to work, you may need to explore other avenues. If you are unable to enjoy the experience, possibly there are other issues that need to be addressed. Seeking outside counsel may be a good next step. They can help you uncover what is really going on. Sometimes we try to fill a void without uncovering the truth first. I am a big believer in getting to the root of problems, not just covering it with a band-aid. Don't give up, just go about it in a different fashion.

SIMPLIFIED AFFIRMATIONS

"My life is filled with passion and purpose"

"I am constantly seeking opportunities to bring about my joy factor"

"I am always willing to make the time for what really matters"

"I am always finding new ways to pursue my passions"

"I am completely supported in creating a life of passion and purpose"

What does life feel like when there is no purpose or meaning? Your life is meant to be enjoyed fully and completely. I am giving you permission to explore your inner guide and follow your heart. We are each born with specific gifts and interests, that is what makes each and every one of us unique in our own way. Some people gravitate towards cleaning up the environment, others lean toward working with the elderly, while others have a passion for working with children and the underpriveleged. Thankfully we each have our own blueprint, so that we have a wide variety of interests and ways to make a difference. Your passion does not have to include feeding the hungry or taking care of the sick. It can be anything and everything that you are naturally drawn to, plain and simple. When you are honoring your passions, you are absolutely making a difference to humanity and contributing to the common good. Explore your passions this week and see where it leads you.

Week 17

Quiet old beliefs and create new ones

We all have beliefs about work, life and ourselves that we bring with us from our upbringing and past experiences. Through our experiences and what people told us growing up, we now look at and embrace life in a certain manner. Possibly your parents told you that you weren't smart enough. Maybe growing up in a large family, you didn't feel like your opinion mattered. These beliefs are limiting in that they are still holding you back from moving forward in your life. *Let me give you an example from a beautiful woman named Julie that I worked with. Julie was a smart, beautiful, warm and sincere individual. Unfortunately she was brought up in a dysfunctional family where her mother went through marriage after marriage. She witnessed the continuous failings of her mother's marriages, so she did not have a positive foundation for a healthy relationship. She assumed all relationships were difficult and petty, and so throughout her own life she experienced turbulent relationships. Because of this upbringing, Julie did not have the belief that healthy and loving marriages were possible. It was not her fault, it was simply the experience that she tapped into.*

On the flip side of negative experiences, are positive and enabling upbringings. Maybe your parents made you feel smart, that you could accomplish anything you set your mind to. Or you witnessed a strong work ethic that is now instilled in you. These beliefs are enabling in that they guide you to be your best. The problem arises when you allow past limiting beliefs to guide your present and future decisions. These limiting beliefs cloud your outlook on life and all that life has to offer.

You do however have the means to create new supportive beliefs, leaving the past where it belongs, in the past. You need to acknowledge that you had no control or choice as to what environment you were raised in. You do have control over your mind and belief system today though. Today can be a fresh start for all you wish to believe. You can also bury all the beliefs that are not benefiting you anymore.

My mother was petrified of death, all the way from a young girl until she eventually passed away. Her father instilled these beliefs in her, and unfortunately she carried them with her for far too long. I wish at the time I could have been more forthright in my own beliefs and convictions. I would have loved to relieve her of her fears and show her that there was nothing to be afraid of. I was too young at the time and didn't have the means to bring up this conversation. I always felt peace regarding the spirituality of death and dying, it was nothing that frightened me. She was very ill at the end of her life, and she probably held on far longer than she should have because of this deep fear. I wish she had the tools to confront her old beliefs and create new, more enriching and supportive beliefs. Sometimes even as adults we have little kids still inside us that need some nurturing and accepting. Realize that some experiences were meant to support and nurture you, and some unfortunately were meant to control and weaken you. This week my advice is to look a little deeper at your past and determine if it is time to create new beliefs and outlooks.

ACTION STEPS FOR THE WEEK:

1. List past beliefs

What did you grow up believing about work, relationships, life and yourself? Take out four pieces of paper and write one of the above words on each piece of paper. I want you to jot down everything you believe about the different areas. Next to these beliefs I want you to write down if the belief is enabling or limiting. Highlight the beliefs that are still limiting you from completely and lovingly moving forward in your life. Let's say for example growing up you were told over and over that you were unattractive. You probably carry this insecurity with you today, and so you have a hard time standing tall and with confidence. This belief is limiting you from having a healthy, balanced and productive life in certain areas.

2. Create new beliefs

Next to each limiting belief, I want you to write down a more positive belief you would like to create and carry with you instead. As a child if you were brought up to believe that all relationships were toxic and unhealthy, you may want to create a new belief system. Possibly writing the words *I am only attracting healthy relationships into my life* may be something you would want to write down. Or you could write *I am surrounding myself by positive and nurturing people.* Write down whatever comes to mind that would be a more positive spin to your current beliefs. You have the power and choice to create whatever beliefs and experiences you want for yourself. No one has the power to choose this for you. I want you to acknowledge this statement and take your control back.

3. Practice makes perfect

Several times a day I want you to read aloud the positive beliefs you created. Focus on the new beliefs until you begin to accept them for yourself. Your thoughts truly become your reality. The art of stating them aloud creates a new belief while replacing the old one. If you focus on the limiting beliefs, you will continue to attract those situations and people to yourself. I want you to bury the old and create some more uplifting beliefs in your life. Practice truly does make perfect. It may take longer for some of you, based on your upbringing and the level of disharmony that you were surrounded by. Just trust that eventually you will be able to leave certain imprints in the past.

One of my most memorable clients was a woman that came to me seeking help moving forward in her life. She had such a sense of humor and warmth about her, that you felt good just in her very presence. Unfortunately she carried a lot of baggage from her upbringing and it affected her in every area of her life. She had weight issues, relationship issues, family conflict, and several more. She had several aha moments in our work together when she finally realized the impact that her negative beliefs were playing in so many areas of her life. She was able to finally confront certain issues and family members who were damaging to her self worth. She felt a huge sense of relief and empowerment. She ultimately took her power back and created an entire new set of beliefs. It completely changed her life. She lost weight,

93

got her finances in order, created healthy boundaries with people, and got back into the dating scene. All of this because she let go of disempowering beliefs that were no longer beneficial to her.

SIMPLIFIED HELP

*I have tried, but I can't seem to get rid of the negative thoughts

Some of you may have more to work with than others. Just remember that it is ok to go at a pace that works for you. Instead of trying to tackle all of your beliefs at once, start with one or two that are the most debilitating. If you are truly having a hard time moving past certain beliefs, don't be afraid to ask for help. Possibly joining a group of individuals that are all tackling the same issues may be beneficial. Getting advice from others and discussing a variety of ways to approach certain situations is great. It helps you look at things from many different angles. Maybe get together a group of close friends and openly talk about ways to confront your negative outlook and beliefs.

*What is the point if I don't really believe the positive beliefs I am stating?

That is exactly why this exercise is so important. The statement *fake it till you believe it* holds true here. Sometimes just the act of faking something over and over, you eventually start to believe it and feel it. Just like my client who faked being extremely confident, eventually she owned those feelings and she was no longer faking. At the beginning you won't believe the statements that you are telling yourself, but over time you will begin to feel a shift. You need to give yourself enough time to really own the new beliefs. If you have had the statement *you are unattractive* in your head for years and years, it may take some time and effort to create a new belief. Don't throw in the towel! It is amazing what can happen when there is consistency and commitment to something.

SIMPLIFIED AFFIRMATIONS

"I have the ability to believe anything I choose"

"My thoughts are my own and only mine"

"I have the strength to release unhealthy beliefs in order to attract loving and nurturing beliefs"

"I am releasing limiting beliefs to the universe"

Write down the beliefs that you are now willing to release:

_____
_____
_____
_____
_____
_____
_____
_____
_____
_____
_____
_____
_____
_____

There are many people who did not experience a supportive, loving and enriching upbringing. Because of this, they spend much of their adult life struggling with inner conflict and resolution. It would have been easy for Oprah Winfrey to assume the world was a dark and difficult existence considering everything she went through as a child. However, she chose at a young age to tap into her inner strength and create her own beliefs and experiences. She completely changed her outlook and saw the good and miracle that life had to offer. She is a direct example of how anyone and everyone can release negative beliefs, and create exactly what they want to believe and experience. You too have the power to make some drastic internal changes if you want it badly enough. Take this week's exercise and begin your own journey of self-exploration.

Week 18

Raise your standards and believe in yourself

Are you fully confident and secure in your own shoes? Do you believe in your own abilities, or do you constantly question who you are as a person? We all have our past, the experiences that shape who we are today. If your past contained lots of criticism, those beliefs don't need to shape your future. Are you tired of being overly critical of yourself and your abilities? There is no better time than the present to start believing in your contributions to those around you. It is so easy to forget everything that you have achieved in your lifetime, because most people focus on what they *lack*, instead of what they excel in.

I worked with Sally after she lost her job. She was extremely down on herself and nervous about searching for a new position. After a couple of weeks, I thought it was time Sally got a fresh perspective on everything she had going for her. I asked her to write down all of her accomplishments and successes in life. At first she laughed at this exercise, but then she took it home and got to work. When I saw her next, we discussed everything on her list. She realized that she had accomplished a huge amount in her life, from professional accolades to personal successes. She started a successful business which she later sold to her partner. She climbed the corporate ladder several times and received significant praise from her superiors. She realized that she always achieved and excelled at whatever she set her mind to. This exercise gave her the visual reminder of the type of person she was. Even though she lost a position, and it was solely due to financial cutbacks, she knew she would be ok. Sally took some time to process everything and she realized she had an opportunity to start fresh and find a job that really excited her. After only two months, she was hired by a company that re-energized her and her outlook. She is happy and blessed to this day. She just needed a reminder of the gifts and talents she brought to the table.

If you do not believe in yourself, how can you expect others to believe in you? If you walked into an interview with your head down and your shoulders hunched over, would you come across as someone confident and self assured? Do you think you would get hired based on this initial assessment? It is important to think highly enough of yourself and your capabilities in order to portray a positive image to others. Each and every one of us is born with special gifts and distinctive traits. Try looking at your life as a whole and piece together everything you have achieved. It is so easy to give credit to others, but for some reason we have a hard time giving ourselves credit where credit is due. I myself used to have a hard time acknowledging everything I do as a mother. I compared myself to my own mother and I felt there was no comparison. My husband and sister had an amazing way of reminding me of my achievements when I needed a little boost. My goal for you this week is to see yourself as others see you. Embrace all that you offer and everything you contribute to those around you.

ACTION STEPS FOR THE WEEK:

1. Review your achievements and successes

I want you to review your life and list all of your achievements. Do not think that this list has to be comprised solely of outstanding achievements. You can write down anything and everything that you view as an achievement. Some examples can be *graduating from college, buying your first home, paying off debt, raising good kids, taking care of a sick relative*, and many more. Do not skip over anything; list as many as you can. If you have a hard time with this exercise, ask your loved ones and friends to help you. Sometimes others have a fresh perspective and can remind you of times you have forgotten. I guarantee that most of you have achieved a lot in your lives, and this is your opportunity to pat yourself on the back and give yourself and emotional boost.

2. Small steps toward success

In order to raise your standards and believe in yourself, you need to embrace self confidence. To feel comfortable with what you have to offer, you have to recall times when you set and achieved goals you set for yourself. This week create some small goals that you can work towards. By setting and then achieving goals, you slowly boost your self confidence and begin to rely on yourself more. After I crossed the finish line of the MS150, I knew that my body was physically capable of whatever challenge I set before it. I tapped into an inner strength that I did not know existed. Every marker you move through will boost your confidence. Make a list of some achievable goals that you would like to attain and then commit to acting on them. Write down your top three:

1.

2.

3.

3. Get rid of your negative self talk

We have discussed this in previous chapters, but it is critically important to your self worth. Every time you think negatively about yourself or others, it lowers your standards. I think holding yourself to a higher standard is important. Don't be the one to gossip or talk down to others; take the high road with class and respect. Wouldn't you feel better about yourself if you were the one that was always positive and respectful towards others? When we talk negatively, it exudes a negative energy toward people. You can literally feel the energy when you meet someone like this. I do not want this to be you. Stand tall and radiate self confidence and positive vibes. It will be in your favor in all elements of your life. Try embracing this concept this week and see how you feel.

SIMPLIFIED HELP

"I know I should raise my standards of myself, but people in my life keep lowering my standards"

I am sure by now you know what I am going to say. You should never give that much power away to anybody else in your life. If someone is lowering the way you feel about yourself, it may be time to release the ties. It is important to surround yourself with people who also have high standards for themselves. This will inspire you to increase your own standards. We feed off each other in both positive and negative ways. If there are people in your life who keep you at a lower standard than you wish for yourself, you need to make some changes. It is hard enough to raise your standards and self worth, but if you are surrounded by people who genuinely want the best for you, it will motivate you to stand tall.

"I can't seem to come up with many achievements in my life"

You are not the first person to have difficulty seeing the positive contributions you have made to the world. Many people are so used to focusing on what is *lacking* in their life, that they do not take the time to acknowledge their successes. If you are having a hard time with this exercise, you need to ask for help from people who know you fairly well. Do you have friends whom you have known for years? Are there family members who will give you honest answers? What about colleagues? Ask them the following questions:
1. What is my greatest accomplishment?
2. What have I achieved in my lifetime?
3. What do I contribute to society?
4. As a young adult or teenager, what hurdles did I overcome?

SIMPLIFIED AFFIRMATIONS

"I am constantly holding myself to a higher standard, being the best I can be"

"I am surrounding myself by people who increase my self-awareness and promote growth"

"I am standing tall and full of confidence"

"I will never allow anyone else to lower my belief in myself"

I worked with Caroline, who struggled with work issues and co-workers who constantly brought her down. Her colleagues were extremely negative in every sense of the word, and it took all of her energy just to avoid them and their distractions. These co-workers obviously had very low standards and felt better when they gossiped about others. When you put forth so much energy talking negatively about people or situations, it automatically lowers your integrity. Try not to fall victim to this trap, it is a very unattractive quality. Caroline eventually realized that this work environment was going to continue to keep her energy low and and her spirits down, so she began looking for a new position. She interviewed and found a position that was not necessarily her ideal job, but the people she would be working with were a refreshing change. They were positive, upbeat, supportive and fun. It made the job exciting and welcoming and she eventually really enjoyed the position and continued to grow into it. This week do what you can to naturally boost your standards and begin the process of believing in yourself and all you have to offer.

Week 19

Say "no" without the guilt

It is amazing how a short word like "no" can cause people so much stress. Most people shy away from saying "no" because they do not want to cause conflict or experience feelings of guilt. I talk with women all the time who wish they could say "no" more, but they can't seem to step outside their comfort zone. How many of you have said "yes" to someone, knowing your true intention and desire was to say "no?" This "yes" leads to more stress and over-obligation. I have a great friend who is exactly one of these people. She is so nice that she says "yes" all the time and then struggles with guilt and the effects of not saying what she would have preferred. She overcommits herself and then stresses that her life is too full and busy. She struggles like so many other women who want to please everyone else, to their own demise. By constantly putting others first, you are not being true to yourself. This week my goal is to help you put yourself and your priorities first. Learn to say "no" and let go of the guilt associated with it.

Jennie struggled with this concept at work. She was the go-to person who took on any project that needed extra work. All of her colleagues would ask her for help or assistance whenever they needed it. They would constantly dump extra work on her desk, and of course she always said "yes" whenever they asked. Knowing that we teach people how to treat us, it was not her colleagues' fault. They got used to Jennie saying "yes", so they relied on her all the time. This caused Jennie to spend many extra hours at the office away from her family. She felt guilty about this, but she did not want to upset anyone at work or let them down. I, of course, mentioned that she was letting her family and herself down by not setting some boundaries. *I asked her to think about what was more important-her family or her co-workers. Obviously her family came first, but she was not acting accordingly. We spent time discussing what she valued most in life and then we embarked on creating a life that honored these values. She eventually was able to respect her time more and she began setting more boundaries at work and with friends. Her life dramatically improved and she felt much better. Her colleagues respected her changes and nothing changed with their relationships. Jennie realized her time was sacred and she wanted to spend it on things that mattered to her. She said "yes" when she really meant it, and she felt ok saying "no" to requests that she didn't want to commit to. She gradually released the guilt and realized that saying "no" was not a hurtful act, but an act of living an authentic life.*

By saying "no" you are not only being true to yourself, but you are respecting everyone who asks something of you. *One of my good friends Dana struggled with this concept. She wanted to please everyone and in the process she was losing a bit of herself along the way. She was constantly trying to come up with excuses for commitments that she wanted to get out of. She did not realize that it would have been much easier and more honest just to say "no" from the beginning. By saying "no" she was allowing the person to find someone who was more excited and able to follow through on the request. Ultimately, this is being authentic with yourself and your time. Dana started practicing saying "no, thank you" and realized that the world did not come to an end. People appreciated her honesty and she felt a huge surge of relief. She said "yes" to requests she genuinely wanted to commit time to and felt better about how she was spending her time.* If you say "yes" just to be nice, chances are you will follow through half-heartedly. This will most likely not go over very well with the person who asked you, and you will not feel very good about yourself either. Only say "yes" if you intend to follow through. This week I want you to decide if some changes need to be made in your own life to get you back on track with what really matters.

ACTION STEPS FOR THE WEEK:

1. Ask for more information

Asking more questions will buy you more time and allow you to weigh your options with your priorities. This will also make it clear to the other person that you are not definitely agreeing to their request at the present time. When someone asks something of you, start by saying *"Let me check my calendar and I will get back to you."* Instead of feeling like you are on the spot to give an answer right away, buy yourself some time. You will feel much more prepared when you get back to them. Ask what the commitment entails and how much time and preparation it will take. Getting answers will help you make your decision.

2. Get your priorities straight

What do you value most in life? Write this down and look at it often. Once you clarify what exactly you want for yourself, it will be easier to stop saying "yes" to things that get in the way. If you value family meals together, but you are volunteering every evening, are you honoring what is most important to you? If you value one-on-one time with your spouse, but your calendar is full of commitments and activities, does this honor what you say is most important? It is crucial to take time every now and then to examine what is most important to you in your life, and then decide if you are living a life that parallels your values. I want you to feel good about how you spend your time. It is ok to say "no" to certain activities, because it may mean a "yes" to someone or something else.

3. Saying "no" is simply refusing the request

You have every right to say "no" without giving a reason. Remember that you are simply refusing the request, not rejecting the person. Most women feel such guilt associated with saying "no" to people because they want to be liked by everyone. Like most anything, the more you practice saying "no," the easier it will become. Your friends, family, and colleagues will respect you much more when you are being honest with your answers. They will also learn to trust that when you say "yes" you really mean it. This week I want you to practice saying "no" and see how it feels. Yes, it may feel awkward at first, but you will feel better being true to your feelings.

I remember working with a client on this topic. Slowly but surely she became more comfortable turning down requests. During this time, I was being interviewed for a TV segment and needed a client to discuss coaching and everything gained from working together. I asked if if she would like to be interviewed by the reporter. She hesitated a minute and then said "no, thank you." She was not comfortable in front of cameras. I was never more proud of a client. I joked with her that she could say "no" to everyone else except for me. She obviously graduated with this lesson deep-rooted.

SIMPLIFIED HELP

"I know I should say 'no' more often, but the guilt lingers way too long"

You are absolutely not alone in your feelings. Typically women want to please everyone and take care of everybody's needs first before their own. In doing this you are chopping away at your spirit little by little. Over time this will wear on you and take its toll. You will harbor negative feelings, guilty feelings, and become overcommitted in the process. We all have a set amount of time in a day and in a week, so it is important to choose wisely how to spend your time. If your guilt lingers too long, then it is important to uncover why this is. Why do you feel like you owe it to others to say "yes?" Are you insecure and so you worry about what they will think? Have you had a hard time setting boundaries for some time? Peel away some layers and start small if need be.

"I am afraid that if I say 'no' at work something bad will happen"

Let me start by saying you absolutely should not say "no" if it is your job to get something done. Do not say "no" if your boss is asking something that is part of your job requirement. I am referring to above-and-beyond expectations. I am referring to colleagues asking you to perform duties that add to your already full work load. If co-workers dump extra work on your desk or ask you to stay late for a project that is not your own, some boundaries need to be drawn. It is ok to let them know that when work is done, you are going to go home to your family. It is acceptable to express that weekends are your time. Just remember that people will respect you more when you are clear on your intentions and honest with your convictions.

SIMPLIFIED AFFIRMATIONS

"I feel comfortable expressing how to best spend my time"

"I am willing and able to say 'no' and everyone is accepting of that"

"By saying 'no' I am essentially saying 'yes' to what really matters"

"I am releasing the guilt associated with saying 'no'"

"I am re-prioritizing how I spend my time with what I value most in my life"

This week is an important one for everyone reading this book. If more of us were honest with how we feel, and we did not do things out of obligation or guilt, life would be less complicated. If you are surrounded by positive and supportive people in your life, they will always accept and care for you even when you decline their invitations. My girlfriends know that I will never get upset if they say "no" to something that I ask of them. We respect each other enough that nobody takes it personally. I, in turn, feel comfortable saying "no" to something if I am simply not in the mood. If this is not the situation for you, there is always room for growth and change. You can talk openly with your friends or family and explain why there is a need for you to set clearer boundaries in your life. Someone needs to pave the way, and I would love for that someone to be you. Start honoring your time and realize that respecting your time will make everything you do commit to more meaningful and full of purpose. Have a great week!

Week 20

Take some much needed "me" time

I am a wife, mother, friend, sister, daughter, volunteer, and business owner. I have a full plate! I have an absolutely wonderful life, but it is demanding and crazy at times. Sometimes the errands, housecleaning, chores and mundane tasks fill every spare moment. I talk with friends and clients all the time who have difficulty setting aside time for themselves. The guilt creeps in like there is no tomorrow. Why do people get so consumed with everyone else's lives, that their own happiness drops to the bottom of the totem pole? By investing in your own life, you are essentially giving a gift to all those around you. When you are happy and at peace, you have so much more to offer. You *can* find a balance between the responsibilities you have taken on, and creating time to nurture yourself. Everyone knows how wonderful it feels to return from a vacation feeling rejuvenated and ready to jump back into life. You do not need to do anything monumental, just commit to taking some time for yourself.

A good friend of mine is a mother of four. Yes, I said four. When we first met she was always frazzled and depleted. She was constantly on the go, acting as a chauffeur for her kids' activities and playdates. She did not set aside time for working out and she was always complaining about it. She has a wonderful husband, but my friend was not accustomed to asking for a lot of help. She figured his main priority was providing for the family and her obligation was taking care of the kids. He was constantly trying to get her to hire more sitters so she could get out of the house every now and then. But she gave in to her guilt and didn't see her "alone" time as a necessity. Well she did not realize her good friend was about to have a chat with her. I typically do not pull out the "life coach card" with friends or family, but this one was different. I was watching my friend drown in the acts of constantly giving to others without giving anything back to herself. I knew she was going to reach a breaking point soon, so I chose to intervene. Looking back now, she could not be more grateful.

I asked her to trust me and try some exercises, and if at the end of it all she did not feel any better, we could go back to the way it was. She hesitantly agreed. We worked on setting boundaries. She began asking for help from friends and her husband. She committed to spending time alone, and ultimately released the guilt associated with making these changes. She began pursuing activities that she put on the backburner for many years. She loved dancing, so she started taking a jazz dance class once a week. She used to meditate regularly, so she began incorporating that into her routine. She woke up earlier in the mornings, before the kids got up, and went for a run. All of these activites brought a calm and peace about her that she had not felt in some time. She realized that nothing drastic needed to change in her family routine, just some basic adjustments. Her husband helped more at night and she hired a regular babysitter. Her friends offered to carpool with her to after school activities. Her kids noticed a shift in their mother and therefore supported her in pursuing activities that brought her joy. She realized the commitment to herself was the most important gift she could give to her kids. The joy she felt radiated to all those around her. Now her children will tell her to take some time to herself if they notice her acting stressed out and restless.

I have always believed that there is no point in working so hard if you are unable to enjoy the benefits. If you were going to drive from Los Angeles to New York, you would need to fill up the gas tank regularly. You would never expect your car to keep going on empty fumes. The same applies to your life. If you go and go but never take the time to fill up your own tank, you will eventually be forced to stop. Aren't you curious why some people get sick over and over again? Maybe they get a cold, then they get a stomach bug, then they fight a migraine, but they keep going. Their body is trying desperately to get their attention. Slow down or you will be forced to slow down.

I have learned over the years how important it is to tune in to my body and nurture it regularly. As soon as I begin to feel as if I am catching something, I force myself to slow down and give my body the much needed rest. In the long run, taking time for myself to decompress and honor my emotional and physical well-being, has benefitted me tremendously. I am blessed to have a husband who pushes me to take care of myself. As soon as he notices that I am stressed out and physically drained, he gently nudges me to take a break. He will entertain the kids, run a hot bath for me, and tell me to go relax. He realizes that by doing this for me, I am much better equipped to take care of the family and everything else going on in our crazy life. Please slow down this week and treat your body and mind with kindness and thoughtfulness.

ACTION STEPS FOR THE WEEK:

1. Be ok with the time

If you are going to set aside time for yourself, you need to feel ok with it. Try letting go of the guilt associated with taking this "me" time. Realize that you are essentially giving a gift to others by taking care of yourself first. When I first had my son, my husband had to coerce me to take a date night. We would go out, but my thoughts were filled with guilt about being home with my son. I simply couldn't allow myself to relax and have fun. After a while I realized how important our date nights were, and I began looking forward to them. I was more relaxed and refreshed, and therefore I had more energy for my son. Guilt simply keeps you from taking care of yourself and your needs.

2. Jot down ideas

What excites you? What would you love to do that you have put off for too long? Jot down everything that brings joy to your life. This list can incorporate simple pleasures as well as more extravagant activities. Do not filter this list, have fun with it. Think back to your past. What do you dream of doing that would put you at ease and bring about peace of mind? For me, doing anything active outdoors is a pure pleasure. Going for a bike ride, taking a hike, enjoying a walk with my husband, or playing sports with my kids brings me joy and bliss. Use the space on the next page to begin your list.

_____
_____
_____
_____
_____
_____
_____
_____
_____
_____
_____
_____
_____

3. Mark it in your calendar and get to work

It is a fact for most people, that if you do not schedule something in your calendar or palm pilot, it will be quickly be forgotten. People are busier than ever, so it is easy to slip your mind. That is why this next step is so important. Looking at the list you compiled, start penciling in activities in your calendar. Make a commitment to yourself that you are important enough to set aside time just for you. You can start with small activities like taking a brisk walk in the morning, or meeting a friend for coffee, seeing a movie by yourself, or simply reading a good novel a little bit every evening. I do not want you to continue reading until you get your calendar out and write some things down! Your life will be that much richer and more joyful when you commit to this time.

SIMPLIFIED HELP

"I have so much going on in my life, I simply do not have the time"

How you spend your time is simply a matter of priorities. My own life is full and busy, however I make the time for myself, not because it is a luxury, but a necessity. If I never take "me" time, I will become drained physically and emotionally. If that happens, I will have nothing to give everyone around me. So, my advice to you is to squeeze in whatever you can. If it means you need to simplify your life a bit first to make some room for what matters, then start with that. But do not put yourself at the bottom of the totem pole, because it will ultimately affect all those around you.

"I am a single parent, so I don't have the support needed to take 'me' time"

Let me start by expressing how much respect I have for single parents. You have a huge responsibility, and I can only presume the difficulties you go through on a daily basis. This is precisely why taking time just for you is even more critical. Sometimes it is a matter of looking outside the box for solutions. Can you ask friends to help with the children? Possibly they can have them over for a playdate on a regular schedule. Perhaps a parent or grandparent can lend a helping hand. Are you able to afford a joint babysitter with another family every so often? This goes back to the guilt of asking for help. Most people, especially friends and family, would be more than willing to offer help when you need it. Remember that this is simply a period of your life that will eventually change. Do what you can now to rejuvenate and refresh your body, mind and spirit.

SIMPLIFIED AFFIRMATIONS

"I will continue to honor myself and my needs"

"Nurturing myself is a priority that I will continue to commit to"

"I am releasing the guilt associated with taking time just for me"

"Cherishing myself and my needs will always benefit others I love"

When my children were seven and four, I trained for my first triathlon. It was very important for me to exercise and get in shape several times a week, if not every day a little bit, and they supported this journey of mine. They saw me train in the pool and wished me luck when I went on long bike rides. When the day of the triathlon came, they were so excited for me because they saw how hard I worked for this day. Crossing that finish line and seeing their faces full of pride and pure joy, made the commitment worth everything. They learned an invaluable lesson that day. They understood that everyone needs time to themselves to relax and decompress. When they are upset or having a difficult day, they also take time to themselves to calm down or just play on their own.

This week try to set aside this essential time for yourself. It may feel awkward or uncomfortable at first, but do not throw in the towel. Give it enough time and effort to really resonate with you in a positive way.

Week 21

Understand past experiences for what they are

Has something ever happened to you, that you did not understand at the time, but as time passed, a reason for the experience revealed itself to you? I am a big believer that everything in your life leads to the next chapter in your life. All of your experiences have led you to exactly where you are today. Whether a situation was difficult, or it was a positive experience, they both led you to this moment...today. In essence, every event is created in your life for a specific purpose. For hypothetical reasons, let us assume you were once in a dead end job, or you lived in an apartment you disliked. What if you met your future spouse while working at the dead end job? Or, you met an extraordinary friend at the apartment complex? Was there an underlying reason for you to be in that exact place at that time in your life? Probably. Many extremely difficult times in my own life have been a catalyst in helping me become the person I am today. Those times have taught me to trust the bigger picture that is coming into focus for each and every one of us.

In my early twenties I was waitressing and figuring out what I wanted to do with my life. This was the same time my mother was extremely ill and needed full-time care. We had several caretakers at her home around the clock, but she always perked up when I walked through the front door. I was very blessed to live very close by, and I spent nine months with her day in and day out. I would comb her hair, play Scrabble with her, feed her through her feeding tube, and spend the night with her in her bed. It was physically and emotionally draining, but I would not change a minute of that period of my life. The time we were able to spend together was priceless and the memories will be with me for the rest of my life. During that time, I would cry myself to sleep every evening and do it all over again the next day. I wanted to be her strength and protector. I honestly did not think I would be able to survive another day, because my heart was constantly breaking into little pieces. Looking back, however, I know I was meant to live close by and have a flexible work schedule so that I could commit most of my time to caring for her. That experience helped me mature into a young woman very quickly. I realized what really mattered to me in life and I vowed to live a wonderful and passionate life in her honor. An inner strength emerged that I did not know existed.

I am a believer that things happen for a reason, typically reasons that are not clearly understood at the time. If you take some time to remember your own past, uncovering reasons why things happened, it may restore your faith in the present. It brings about a peace of mind that things will always work out the way they are supposed to. I do not worry as much now when things happen. I have faith that there is a reason behind everything, and I now release worry and anxiety to the universe. Sometimes we try so hard to understand why something is happening, and the reason may not unveil itself until you are ready to receive it.

I worked with a woman who had completely hit rock bottom in her life. She lost her job, she was extremely overweight, and her husband recently left her for her best friend. I know this sounds like a ficticious story, but it was her life. At the time, there was no way she was going to understand why everything was happening to her. After working together for four months or so, her life completely turned around. She found a job that she absolutely loved, one that she never thought would fall into her lap. She started a weight loss program and lost twenty pounds. And, she started dating wonderful men who found her exciting and fun. Looking back, had she not lost her job, she would never have found the position she currently holds. She is passionate about this job and expresses gratitude every day she wakes up for the opportunity. She also acknowledges that her husband was not a great fit for her, she deserved someone more attentive and affectionate. She realized that everything in her life happened for a specific reason and she is blessed to have had the ability to move past the difficult times with faith. Her life is full of joy and purpose, all because she did not hide under a rock and accept her fate for what it was.

This week open yourself up to the prospect that things in life happen for a reason. You may not understand or come to terms with why certain things happen, but have faith that you will appreciate everything at a later date. I know how difficult it is to release the stress and anxiety when you are going through challenging times. I have conquered many difficult times in my own life, but it is much easier to move through these times when you have an understanding of the bigger picture. I know the universe is always on my side and that I will be protected when I most need it. Try incorporating these tips this week and see how your outlook changes.

ACTION STEPS FOR THE WEEK:

1. Review your past

I want you to review your past experiences, the ones that were particularly difficult at the time. Are you able to uncover the reasoning behind them? Can you now see why certain things happened? Did someone ever come into your life the exact time you needed them? *I met my husband in January of 1995. At the time my mother was terminally ill and the last thing on my mind was meeting men. The universe had other plans for us though. We quickly fell in love and he was my rock during the most painful and difficult time in my entire life. I do not think I would have survived without him by my side. His mother was also terminal, so I was able to support him through his own nightmare. Looking back, I am so grateful that we met at the exact time we needed each other the most.* Jot down why you think certain experiences presented themselves to you.

Event   *Why it happened?*

2. Your present life

Now that you have reviewed your past, what challenges are you currently dealing with? Are you unhappy with certain elements of your life? Is there a positive spin you can make out of your current situation? Remember that you may not be able to see the full picture right now, and it may take some time for the truth to be unveiled. Just have faith that you are where you need to be right now. When I am worrying about something going on in my life, just taking a step back and thinking positively will instantly shift my mood. I know that stress and anxiety will not change anything, other than put me in a depressed state of mind, so I try to release it. If you are currently struggling with some challenges in your own life, can you try to visualize a positive end result? It is amazing what a shift in our thinking can do to the big picture.

3. Don't settle

Just because you have faith in the bigger picture, does not mean you have to settle for things that make you unhappy. Are you unhappy in a relationship? Are you dissatisfied with work? Fate will step in when it needs to, but in the mean time take control of your life and the choices you make. I am a firm advocate in not settling in life for things that make you unhappy. As you are facing challenges, you can both release the stress and anger, and be proactive at the same time. Take ownership for moving forward in your life and have faith that you are being supported along the way. If you find yourself settling often in your life, it may be time to take a step back and do what it takes to enhance your self worth.

I remember very vividly when the September 11th tragedy happened. It shook my foundation to the core. I was in shock, deeply depressed, scared, and highly emotional in every area of my life. My son was only one at the time and I was afraid of the world he was being brought up in. I questioned everything and wanted to hang on to everyone in my life very tightly. It took quite a bit of time to move through the fog and uncertainty, but eventually I used this experience as a significant catalyst in my life. I did not take anything for granted. I became more engaged in the time I spent with my son and husband. I was instantly more compassionate with others who were struggling in their own lives.

I appreciated every little thing that life had to offer, and I had a renewed sense of being blessed. I never could understand why so many lives had to be lost, but I was able to create some good from a very unfortunate and heartbreaking experience. If I am able to love more completely, and make a positive difference in people's lives, then some good has come from an unimaginable tragedy.

SIMPLIFIED HELP

"I cannot possibly see any good from the bad experiences in my life"

When I am discussing negative experiences in your life, I am not referring to all experiences. Every experience is different, and some incidents may be too difficult to discuss. I would like to talk about the majority of negative things that happen in our lives. If you went through difficult break-ups, did you tap into a strength you did not know existed? Did you come to realize more clearly what type of partner you were looking for? If you struggled financially as a child, did you adopt a healthier attitude when it comes to finances? Are you now committed to saving money and putting aside funds for a rainy day? I want you to see that you can always see the silver lining if you look hard enough.

"I have too much anger and sadness to see the positive side of things"

You may either be too close to the memory to see it in a different light, or you may need support moving past the anger. If you are consumed with resentment, you will stay stuck in that period. You are not fully free to move on with your life. Can you work on forgiveness from either someone else or yourself? Are there different ways to look at the situation? My advice would be to bring on the support of someone who can move you from pain to freedom. Research a therapist, counselor, life coach, or clergy member to be your partner. Journaling is also a great tool to help you put all of your feelings in a safe place.

SIMPLIFIED AFFIRMATIONS

"I trust that there is always a bigger picture playing out for me"

"There is always a purpose for everything that happens in my life"

"I accept that people and situations will always come into my life when I need them"

"I am always protected and guided in my life"

One of my clients was devastated when her boyfriend of two years decided it was time to part ways. She assumed she would marry this man, and she was completely mystified by his desire to leave. She felt as if she would never meet anyone as special, and her self esteem dropped quite a bit. It took a while for her to get re-engaged in her life, but slowly I started to see the spark in her eyes again. She took time to nurture herself and take care of her needs, something I always recommend to people who have just lost a significant relationship. After the initial shock, she was able to see the relationship from a different perspective. She realized it was not as perfect as she once thought it was. Something very important to her was having a partner who was as adventurous as she was. She loved to travel and see different cultures, and her boyfriend preferred to stay at home and relax. She needed to be with someone who also had a desire to see the world and visit other cultures. She recognized that she sacrificed a lot throughout this relationship. She finally had an interest to meet someone that was a better life match and she created peace with her ex-boyfriend.

This week is about coming to terms with the fact that things tend to happen for a reason and trusting this will make your life a little bit easier. Good luck!

Week 22

Valuable lessons in challenging yourself

How often do you really challenge yourself? This could involve your career, personal challenges, physical challenges, or any combination. I have started a tradition with some girlfriends of doing something physically challenging every summer. It started with a triathlon, and last year I completed a 150-mile bike ride. For me, life is not meant to be without risk and adventure. My father has always been a wonderful role model in this belief. He always challenges himself and explores new things, a wonderful quality that I hope to instill in my own life. I think it is important to raise the bar every now and then and surprise yourself with achievements that you would not normally give yourself the opportunity to try. Life becomes very humdrum and monotone if you do not venture out every now and then. How do we grow and evolve as individuals if we do not ever push ourselves past our comfort zones? I never once thought I would be able to ride 150 miles on my bike in two days. The fact that I tried something I thought was way past my capability, and actually accomplished it, was a huge feat. Another example came on the morning of my triathlon. I saw women of every size, shape and age. It was so humbling to see all these individuals achieve something that society might label only fit for specific body types and ages. There was a woman in her mid-fifties and blind who beat my time by over an hour. I could not have been more inspired.

I have a good friend who was always nervous in social situations. She was such a joy, but she was a bit insecure when it came to parties and get togethers. I asked her what would be the scariest thing she could think of doing, and she said speaking in front of a group. She always had this fear and it held her back in so many ways. We came up with a way for her to challenge herself in this arena and break the mold that had been there for so long. She signed up for an improv class at a local theater. This was completely out of her comfort zone, but she was open to the task. After a couple of months, she felt completely liberated. She realized once she got over the initial fear of being the center of attention, she actually got a rush of energy. Everyone in her class was completely supportive and gentle with her, and she was able to shed a fear that consumed her throughout her life. She was then able to go to parties and get involved in conversations without a second thought. She completely amazed herself and her husband with her newfound confidence. I was so proud of her and loved watching her evolve over time. The fact that she was willing to challenge herself in this way taught her that she was much stronger and more resilient than she ever thought.

Are there opportunities in your own life where you could push the bar a bit higher? Are there ways where you know you could challenge yourself, but the fear is holding you back? For me, writing this book was a huge challenge in so many ways. To start with, I did not know the first thing about the process of writing a book. I had to research and learn the order of creating a book from start to finish. The commitment to write when I had a million and one other things to get done, was a steep learning curve for me. The creation of this book has opened my eyes to so many life lessons. If you want something in your life bad enough, you -and only you- can do what it takes to bring it to fruition. No matter what the outcome of this book is, and how many lives it is able to change positively, I will be proud that I challenged myself physically and mentally to bring it to life. This book will be a wonderful legacy and tool for my children when they are old enough to understand and embrace the concepts. This week is about taking a look at your own life and determining if there are specific areas where you can push yourself a bit. Try to look outside the box and do not limit yourself to what you think you can do. I guarantee each and every one of you reading this book can do something that you thought you were never capable of doing. However, you need to give yourself the opportunity to try, or you will never know.

ACTION STEPS FOR THE WEEK:

1. Is your life "comfortable?"

Do you feel there is little excitement in your life? Do you feel an urge to try new things? Are you becoming restless? These questions will determine whether or not you need to push yourself and challenge yourself. You may be feeling a void, you may feel a lack of direction, or you may constantly wish for more in your life. If you are aware that there is little enthusiasm or enjoyment in your life, now is the time to move past that. Remember that nobody can do this for you, there has to be an internal desire to make some changes. If you feel your life is fairly monotonous, move on to step number two.

2. What is calling out to you?

Have you always dreamed of running a marathon? Are you itching to put your name in the running for a promotion? What have you given thought to in the past or present, that you have not acted on? Jot down what ideas come to mind. Remember it can be physical challenges, mental challenges, professional challenges, or a mix of the above. Think outside the box here. Do not limit yourself- have fun with this list. This is just the beginning of your journey, and the list will continue to expand as time goes on. Place a star next to the challenges that call out to you the most. These are the ones you may want to go after first.

_____

_____

_____

_____

_____

_____

_____

_____

_____

_____

_____

_____

3. **Move forward**

Now that you have an idea of the challenges you want to embark on, it is time to take action. Ideas are futile if there is no action. Even if you are simply taking baby steps, you are doing more than you were doing before. Do not beat yourself up if you do not move at a fast pace. Just break down the challenges you came up with above into bite size steps. Let's take, for example, that you want to climb a fourteen-thousand-foot mountain. Does this seem out-of-character or a far-fetched goal? What can you do so it doesn't seem so daunting? Pick a date that you would like to climb the mountain. How can you prepare yourself physically? Some examples would be to hire a trainer, hike smaller trails, and build up your endurance. Write down some smaller goals in your calendar that will move you forward, closer toward your end result. The only things holding you back are self-defeating thoughts or behaviors. There is always a way, you just need to get creative and open your mind. Get going!

One client who stands out was a woman in her mid- thirties. She was full of life and passion. She separated from a boyfriend and came to realize that she had never really been alone in her adult life. She was constantly going from boyfriend to boyfriend, and in the process she was stepping further away from her authentic self. She did not know who she was or what her likes were, because she was so used to putting men first. A big challenge and discomfort for her was to remain single for a lengthy period of time. She knew she needed to do this in order to regain self- respect and remember what really mattered to her. She needed to get re-acquainted with the woman she saw in the mirror. So, she accepted the challenge to remain single until she felt she was healthy in body, mind and spirit. She came to realize that being single was not as scary as she envisioned it would be. She looked forward to spending time with friends, organizing her home, and getting involved again in exercise and meditation. She treasured this challenge and after six months slowly ventured back into the dating scene. She had a newfound approach however, and knew that she did not need a man to complete her. She was simply looking for someone to enjoy her life with.

SIMPLIFIED HELP

"I like feeling safe and secure where I am"

I respect and honor where you are in your life. If you are ok with your life "as is" and do not feel the need to challenge yourself, then that is completely your choice. All of the tips and advice in this book are to be taken with a grain of salt. You will connect with some of the tips and not others, and that is fine. I think it is wonderful to feel safe and secure where you are in life, but you can still feel safe while slowly venturing toward unchartered territory. The wonderful thing is that you can explore and challenge yourself at your own leisure and see how you feel. It may open something up in you that you then choose to explore deeper. Or, you may decide that you are completely at peace with where you are. The choice is yours to make, and you can always change your mind.

"I am afraid I will fail if I challenge myself"

Do you know what my belief is on failure? You will absolutely, unequivocally never fail as long as you try. If you give something your best and you "fail," then it simply was not meant to be. What do you gain by "failing?" You are able to stand tall and confident in the knowledge that you tried something new and unfamiliar. You gain so much more self respect when you try, no matter what the outcome. This is a concept I constantly express to my clients. Even if you do not succeed in the manner that you first envisioned, you will succeed in so many other ways. My advice is not to be so preoccupied with the end result. Just give it your all and reap the rewards.

SIMPLIFIED AFFIRMATIONS

"I am open to the challenges that are presented to me"

"I am constantly seeking to evolve and grow as a person"

"I know that challenging myself will act as a catalyst toward boosting my self esteem and self image"

"I commit to taking risks and seeing where they lead me"

"I have faith that I will survive any challenge that comes my way"

Because I am such a believer in challenging yourself, I am constantly seeking new challenges in my own life. Some may revolve around my career, some focus on physical challenges, and some may emphasize challenging myself mentally. I have gotten attuned to noticing when my life feels complacent. I used to meditate every day before I had children. Once my kids came into my life, and free moments were few and far between, meditation got lower and lower on my priority list. Eventually meditation was a distant memory. I chose to create my own challenge. No matter how tired I was, or how many other pressing responsibilities I had, I was determined to get up early every morning and meditate. Trust me when I say that this was one of the more difficult challenges I embarked upon. I knew once I got started and it became part of my daily routine, the challenge would slowly dissipate. I feel so much clearer in every area of my life when I take the time to meditate. It is a valued part of my day now. So, my wish for you this week is to come up with ways you can challenge yourself. Remember there is no wrong way to complete this exercise. Simply decide whether or not you need to push out of your self imposed box and try new things. I have complete confidence that each and every one of you can do so much more than you believe you can; you just need to try.

Week 23

When life throws you a surprise

How many of you thought things were going pretty smoothly in your life, when all of a sudden life threw you a curve ball? There were many times when things were going my way, and then the unexpected happened. Possibly you lost a job, or a relationship suddenly ended, or a good friend betrayed you. How you react to these curve balls makes all the difference. This is when your strength of character and positive outlook will act as a compass to guide you forward. When unexpected things happen to you, it is important to embrace your feelings, rely on a supportive group of friends, and have faith that you will survive this chapter in your life. I have mentioned several times before in this book, I am a believer in learning life lessons as you go, so that the universe does not continue to send you similar lessons. Sometimes there is a lesson to be learned, and sometimes something unfortunate simply happens that you have no control over.

Due to the economy, one of my clients lost a high- paying corporate position. Understandably at first, he was completely thrown off course. He had been at this position for quite some time, and had grown comfortable with the lifestyle and perks. Something he never got used to however, was his lack of involvement with his children's lives. He worked long hours and traveled quite a bit. Although this provided very well for his family, it took its toll. All of a sudden, life pulled the rug out from under him. After taking some time to process everything, he decided to take this opportunity to spend quality time with his wife and children. They had plenty in savings so there was no rush to jump back in right away. We discussed his many options and he eventually decided that he wanted to start his own consulting business. He had plenty of contacts and colleagues to connect with, and this would give him the flexibility and ability to work from home. He never would have taken this leap had the universe not stepped in. He discovered a newfound excitement in his career, and his family loved seeing him more. When he lost his job, he was clearly at a fork in the road. He could have seen this unfortunate curve ball as a horrible situation that left him a victim to circumstances. Or, he could have used this situation as a catalyst to create something positive. He chose to create something positive from an unfortunate event in his life. Whether you disagree with what life throws your way or not, becoming a victim will only keep you at that point.

This chapter is especially important, because you will always encounter curve balls in your life. Life will constantly throw roadblocks your way to see how you react and evolve from them. Watching my mother suffer could have made me very bitter and hopeless. It would have been easy to believe life was not fair and thus trigger me to be blinded to the many gifts and blessings in my life. I went through a period of wanting to escape everything, wishing I could stay in bed all day every day. Luckily, I was surrounded by friends who helped me see the light through a very dark and confusing tunnel. We all have choices as to how we are going to respond to unexpected curve balls. If you believe in yourself and your ability to bounce back, you will always come out stronger and more resilient.

I have witnessed the unfortunate way people can unravel when they cannot bounce back from an unforeseen event. Many people will turn to food, alcohol or drugs to cope. This is sad to witness because all of those coping mechanisms are short-lived and detrimental to your physical and mental health. Most of these crutches act as a band-aid, helping you feel good right away, but fail to improve you long-term. If you have a pattern of turning to food, alcohol or drugs when life surprises you, I would advise seeking treatment from a trained therapist. You can always find great information at the Psychology Today (www.psychologytoday. com) website. This resource can help you break this self destructive behavior and give you the tools to make healthier choices. This chapter will help you create a protective layer so you are better equipped to deal with something when, and if, it comes your way.

ACTION STEPS FOR THE WEEK:

1. Review your past

Are there similar curve balls that continue to pop up in your life? Is there a pattern that has developed? If so, realize that the common denominator may be *you*. For example, if you have been divorced four times and are constantly surprised when your spouse leaves you, there may be an underlying issue that needs to be addressed. What can you take responsibility for so it does not continue to happen? Blaming others and feeling like a victim will only go so far. Of course there are times when you do not control a situation, but my goal is to help you see other patterns that you may be able to break. I want you to be the driver in your life, not the passenger. I want you to learn from your past so that you can ultimately change the course of your future.

2. When have you persevered?

Sometimes when life throws us a surprise, we feel completely ill-equipped to handle the situation. We feel powerless and unsure how to move forward. Occasionally you just need a reminder that you can face any adversity or situation that comes your way. Reviewing your life up to now, when did you face a difficult challenge? Did you survive? Did you somehow manage to tap into a strength you did not know existed? Write down every single situation that you can recall when you overcame a difficult time in your life, and look at this list often. When another challenge comes your way, pull out this list and remind yourself that you are a survivor and can handle whatever hand you are dealt.

Experience	*What you did to survive*

3. Brainstorm healthy coping mechanisms

We all need ways to cope with stressful situations. Every single one of us is unique in that we respond differently to trauma and anxiety. Personally, I thrive on alone-time and the outdoors. Whenever I feel stressed or worried about something, I know what will bring me peace of mind. If I can listen to music, meditate, journal, take a hot bath with a cup of tea, go for a brisk walk, or take my bike out for a relaxing ride, I will always feel calmer. This time allows me to process everything going on, and because I am able to clear my mind, I always come up with solutions and avenues to tackle the situation. Over time, I have created my own list of coping mechanisms that help me face whatever curve ball is thrown my way. I want you to brainstorm your own list of ways to cope with the unexpected. Come up with anything and everything that will bring you peace, both mentally and physically. Keep this list handy so you can rely on it whenever you need helpful ideas.

Healthy coping mechanisms:

_____

_____

_____

_____

_____

_____

_____

_____

SIMPLIFIED HELP

"Every time life throws me a curve ball, I cannot seem to get past it"

I realize that there are many different levels of curve balls. Some are fairly minor and easy to overcome, while others rock our world. If you are feeling fragile in that you do not have faith that you can face adversity, I would start with that. What can you do to feel more capable? What did you do in the past that helped you move through difficult times? Do you have friends who seem to always face challenges with a positive outlook? Talk with them and try to discover what works for them.

"Why do some people get bombarded with life lessons, while others breeze by?"

I absolutely believe that some people seem to attract more hurdles in their lives than others. This all goes back to attitude and your general outlook on life. If you assume you will always have a difficult and complicated life, then you probably will. If, on the other hand, you have a positive approach to life, you will be more likely to move past challenging situations. You will more than likely attract fewer difficulties. Everyone will be dealt hard times every now and then, but it is how you react to these hardships that make all the difference. Try not to be too consumed with other people, just focus on yourself and have faith that you will persevere through whatever life throws at you.

A client named Grant came to see me after he had a huge health scare. He was rushed to the hospital and diagnosed as having suffered a minor heart attack. Up to that point, Grant did not live a very healthy lifestyle. He smoked regularly, drank often, traveled quite a bit for work, did not exercise, and had a negative outlook on life. He was simply a walking time bomb. After his heart attack, Grant had two choices as to how to proceed. He could have ignored the universe's nudge and continued living his life the way he was accustomed to. Or, he could take the heart attack as a very clear sign to make some lifestyle changes. Thankfully he came to see me at the exact right time. He was a smart man and realized that he was given a second chance to finally make some adjustments. He knew that if he did not use his heart attack as a wakeup call, he probably would not be alive for long. Grant completely turned his life around and is proof that sometimes you just need a little motivation to get back on track.

SIMPLIFIED AFFIRMATIONS

"I have faith that I can survive any challenge that comes my way"

"I am secure in my ability to persevere through any difficulty"

"I am always protected and guided by the universal light energy"

"I will always tap into an inner strength to get me through difficult situations"

How many of you reading this chapter have encountered challenges in your life? I would bet the majority of you have faced adversity. Most of these experiences have made us stronger and more resilient. Work on becoming more aware of this concept this week. Know that life will continue to place hurdles in your way, but you have the power to jump over these hurdles. There are people who feel more comfortable playing the "victim" role, and they will define themselves as victims throughout their life. Because of this, the universe will continue to throw experiences their way to validate their belief. If, on the other hand, you genuinely believe that you can handle anything that comes your way, you will create a protective shield around yourself. You will still have to face hardships in your life, but you will get through them much faster and with more ease. Thank you for having faith in the bigger picture this week. It will always steer you in the right direction.

Week 24

eXamine whether to stay in a relationship or go

Over the years, I have talked with countless individuals who were torn about whether to stay in a relationship or move on. One woman in particular had been with her boyfriend for seven years. She was fairly unhappy and did not know whether to keep working at it or let it go. There were many key issues that continued to pop up over the years, but she never had the strength to end it for good. She knew deep down he was a good man, but in her heart she felt she was meant to be with someone else. I need to emphasize that there is no magic formula for whether one should stay or go. Whether you are unhappily married, or in a committed relationship that lacks passion, it is an individual decision that should not be taken lightly. You never want to base a decision out of fear, unless it is real physical or mental fear. By this I mean that you should not stay in something only because you are afraid of being alone. Or, you should not commit to someone because you are afraid you will never find anyone else.

Ideally, you want to be with someone for the right reasons. You need to be compatible, genuinely like each other, have similar values and visions of the future, and respect and honor one another. Every relationship is going to have its ups and downs. You cannot expect to always get along. If you are in a situation where you are going back and forth on whether to stay or leave, it is important to take a step back and examine the relationship from a fresh perspective. Remember that if two people are committed to making things work, and they still love each other as partners and friends, they have a great chance of growing as a couple. Also keep in mind that there may be a time when, as a couple, you have exhausted your efforts and may be ready to part ways.

Rhonda was married for nineteen years. She and her husband had three children and a beautiful home. Even though on the outside, they looked like the perfect couple, she was unhappy and unfulfilled in the marriage. Once we got down to the real issues, she admitted she had been unhappy most of their marriage. She felt trapped and uncertain on what to do. She stayed in the marriage for the kids and the lifestyle, but it was getting to the point where the unhappiness was taking a physical and mental toll on her. She knew she was staying for the wrong reasons, but she feared being on her own. She was so accustomed to being the wife and mother, that she lost her own identity over the years. Her children were old enough to not only take care of themselves but to understand that their mother needed to do what would ultimately make her happy. She knew that this marriage did not enhance her in any way, it depleted her. After working together for a while, she gained the strength and awareness to do what she needed to do. Her husband inherently knew this day was coming and surprisingly supported her decision.

This chapter is about helping you make a difficult decision in order to enrich your life. I believe that each and every one of us deserves to be respected and unconditionally loved in a relationship. Any relationship will take work and commitment on both parties, but it should not feel like you are constantly swimming upstream. If there is a lot of drama, a lot of fighting, disrespecting of either person, and a genuine lack of affection, you may want to listen to those red flags as warning signs. If you are constantly making excuses as to why your partner is not treating you very well, you may want to look at that as well. We teach others how to treat us, so make sure you expect to be treated with kindness and respect. This week is about uncovering the truth so that you feel comfortable making a decision.

ACTION STEPS FOR THE WEEK:

1. Happy or unhappy?

Are you or are you not currently happy in your relationship? Is your partner also dissatisfied? Are you constantly looking to your partner to make you happy? Asking someone else to provide your happiness is a huge request to ask of any one person. Remember that just because you are not happy, does not mean there is anything critically wrong in your relationship. You may need to focus on getting involved in activities that bring more joy to your life. You could be blaming your partner for your unhappiness, when you need to take responsibility for creating your own happiness. It may simply not be about them.

On the flip side of the coin, there may be fundamental problems that need to be addressed. If you are very satisfied and happy in all the other areas of your life, except for your relationship, then clearly this is the part that needs some attention. If you have been unhappy for quite some time, and your partner is not interested in working to improve the relationship, it may be time for you to explore your options. I am a believer in the 90-10 rule. You should be happy and at peace with your partner ninety percent of the time. The other ten percent of the time you are going to have disagreements and difficult periods to work through. If on the other hand you are happy ten percent of the time, but you argue and fight ninety percent of the time, it would be best to part ways.

2. Time to be proactive

If there are fundamental problems in your relationship, have you sought out help? I commend couples who reach out for help when they do not know where to turn. This means they still have the fight and desire to make things work. If you still care for your partner, do not throw in the towel before you have given it your all. No matter the final outcome, you will feel at peace that you gave it your best effort. This takes both people wanting to make things work. If only one person in the relationship is invested in this process, then it will be difficult to move forward. This week determine how committed you both are to improving your relationship. If you are both on board, seek out some help from a therapist or relationship coach. If either one of you is ready to move on because you do not have the desire to work things out, it may be time to have a conversation. It does not mean either one of you failed, or that your relationship was a failure, it simply means you were probably not meant to be together. I believe every relationship is meant to serve a specific purpose. You grow and evolve as people, whether the relationship was positive or toxic. Even if you are leaving an unhappy relationship, you now know more clearly what you are looking for, and you are hopefully standing taller and stronger for the experience. Try seeing the positive in every situation.

3. Do not let fear be the decision maker

If you are extremely unhappy in a relationship and you have tried several methods of reconciliation, then it may be time to take a break. So many people assume it is a black or white issue, meaning you either stay together or completely break up. There is always gray area to explore if you choose. One choice is to temporarily separate in order to re-think your options and see how it feels to be alone. Do not let fear be the sole deciding factor. If you are simply afraid of being alone, afraid of never finding another partner, or afraid of exploring life by yourself, that may not be a good enough reason to stay. Each and every one of you is stronger than you may think. Make sure you either leave for the right reasons or stay for the right reasons.

A dear friend of mine was at a point in her marriage where she thought hard about leaving her husband. He had been unfaithful to her and this was the ultimate betrayal. She vowed she would never stay with someone who cheated on her, but this time was different. They had two small children to consider. She went back and forth on what to do, and luckily her husband made it clear that he would do whatever it took to save the marriage. He was completely committed to seeking a therapist and putting the pieces back together. It took quite some time, but they were ultimately able to move forward and create some healing. It has been ten years and they are still happily married and very grateful that they did not give up too quickly on the marriage. Because they were both invested in saving the family, they were able to heal the marriage and move on.

SIMPLIFIED HELP

"We are perfect for each other except for one small detail"

One small detail for one person is a big deal for someone else. You need to define how important this small detail is in the big picture.

Maybe you get along wonderfully but when your partner is upset he gets emotionally abusive. Possibly you have found the perfect woman except for the fact that she is still very friendly with all of her ex-boyfriends. Is your small detail something that can be fixed? Is your partner willing to improve the relationship in that area? Only you can decide whether or not this "small detail" is going to continue to degrade your relationship. Stick to your values and do not compromise. Everything else can be addressed and improved if both partners have the desire.

"I honestly do not think I can make it on my own"

Let me start by saying that every situation is unique. If there are financial reasons why you feel the need to stay, it may not be realistic to jump ship just yet. Possibly you need to do some research and begin saving money for a rainy day. The fact that you are investing time and energy in this book says a lot. You have the tools and know-how to make a change. However, if you feel incapable in some way, reach out for help. I do not believe anyone should be miserable in a relationship. I want you to be in the drivers seat and feel comfortable being in control of your happiness. Do what you can to boost your confidence. Read books, talk with people and see what options you have at your disposal.

SIMPLIFIED AFFIRMATIONS

"I am in a loving and committed relationship"

"I am beautiful and worthy of an enriching relationship"

"I have the tools to create a respectful and loving partnership"

If you are confused and unsure what to do with a relationship, sometimes you just need to take a step back and gain some fresh perspective. *A client, Carol, kept going back and forth trying to decide whether to leave her boyfriend. She loved him dearly but none of her friends or family approved of him. He was a musician and did not have dreams of living a corporate and reliable lifestyle. Carol loved his creativity but she also worried about his ability to provide for a family when they had one. After discussing her values and what was most important to her, she realized she needed security in her life. She came to terms with the fact that her boyfriend might not be the best husband material for her. She would always care for him as a person, but she did not envision them creating a life together. Her boyfriend would always live a more laid back lifestyle and he also did not want to feel forced to be someone he was not. It was a mutual decision to part ways.* This week I want you to take some quiet time to reflect on your dilemna. Make sure whatever decision you ultimately make comes from your values, not from fear. Continue the great work!

Week 25

You deserve a job you love, get out there!

How many of you feel stuck in a job that does not excite or inspire you? Are you staying put for security and comfort? Do you dread the thought of being there five years from now? If this sounds familiar, it may be time to shift your thinking. If you are a passenger in the car that is navigating through your life, then you are simply going along for the ride. I want you to sit in the driver's seat. I want you to oversee the direction and ultimate destination of your life. One main component is your career. Your career takes up a large majority of your time, whether full-time or part-time. Life is far too short to go through the motions for the sake of "getting through" another day. Wouldn't you love to wake up excited about the day that lies before you?

Early on in my marriage, my husband and I were both at a crossroads in our careers. We decided to get involved in real estate and create a business working together. My husband naturally gravitated toward home improvements; he could fix anything, spruce things up, and he had a wonderful eye for what makes a house a home. So, we decided it would be a lucrative profession that we could share as a couple. We studied and passed the exam and became licensed real estate professionals. At the beginning we had a great time working together and sharing in the responsibilities. I knew fairly quickly that this was clearly not the career path for me. The emotional strain that I took on from clients wore me down. I was miserable and it took a physical toll on me. I was not sleeping well and I simply disliked the business. My husband, on the other hand, loved the profession and was extremely good at it. He had a natural ability to connect with clients and offer them superior service. They loved him and consistently referred him to friends and colleagues. I knew a difficult discussion was on the brink.

I knew intuitively that this was not my path in life and I shared with him that I needed to explore other options that were more up my alley. He was sad that we would not be able to continue working together in the way that he envisioned. He wanted me to be happy though, so he supported my decision. And, he thrived in business once I left his side. He was able to work in a fashion that worked for him, without worrying about me as his partner. He created his own system and continues to have a very busy and successful real estate business to this day. I am so proud of him and all that he has accomplished. He followed his own strengths and passions and created a career out of something he naturally enjoys.

Some of you may have lost jobs due to the economy and some of you simply may be unhappy where you are. This chapter is important so that you can find a position that taps into your strengths and natural passions. If you are able to find a job that is fulfilling to you, you will be very blessed. Many people get caught up in the routines of a job they dislike and do not take the time to explore other options. This week is about taking some time to reflect on what you enjoy while exploring your professional past.

ACTION STEPS FOR THE WEEK:

1. Past and present

What experiences in your past made you feel the most alive? Review previous jobs and experiences so that you can begin to map out a future. What skills have you acquired over the years? What can you bring with you to your next position? Write down memories from when you felt the most alive. For example, digging in the dirt, speaking at a ceremony, volunteering for Habitat for Humanity, or working with kids. All of these memories act as a blueprint for what you are naturally drawn to. These are the clues to get you started. Also write down all the skills you have acquired. For example, accounting, organizing, speaking, delegating, or researching- this is all expertise to highlight on your resume.

Memories   **Skills**

_____
_____
_____
_____
_____
_____
_____
_____
_____
_____

2. Expand your thinking

Part of this process is opening your mind to all possibilities. Do not hold back. What would you love to explore? What are you excited just thinking about? Create a visual "collage" of what an ideal job would look like. I want you to purchase a piece of poster board and tap into your creative side. What would you be doing? Who would you surround yourself by? Where are you? Get out magazines, markers, paint, or simply a pen or pencil. Cut out pictures illustrating your dream job. Cut and paste or just write down your vision. This vision board is the beginning of manifesting your ideal position. You cannot go after something that you have not thought about first. Do not filter this dream job, just see what comes up when you let your mind go.

3. Be realistic

If you are unhappy at work, it is not a good idea to quit your job today and simply embark on your passions. This is about planning for your future and doing the necessary research first. Do you need a financial safety net before you move forward? Do you need to discuss your options with family members first? I am a firm believer in educating yourself, doing research and then planning accordingly. I want you to make rational and well thought-out decisions. How can you set yourself up to succeed? How can you create a specific time line to move you forward? Come up with realistic goals that you can work toward. Set specific dates so you have markers to reach for. If you would like to leave a job within six months, detail exactly what needs to happen for this to be an achievable goal. The more specific you are the more likely it is that you will achieve your desired result.

When Dani came to see me she was struggling with her current employer. She was extremely dissatisfied and unfulfilled, but she did not know how to cut the ties. She was extremely gifted as a gardener and she absolutely loved creating flower vases and putting together gifts for friends. She had a natural knack for it. This was the one area of her life that brought her pure joy and peace of mind. She was working at a company where it was all about numbers and sales. She was not tapping into her stengths, and it was very clear to me why she was so unhappy. We devised a plan to move her closer to her dream of becoming a respected florist. We picked a date exactly one year from the time we began working together. In that time, she was going to take floral arrangement classes, volunteer time with a florist she knew, save money, pay off debt, and take some business classes. We had a very specific timeline for her to follow and she felt much better about the prospect of leaving her job. Because she knew exactly what she needed to do, and she had the support to keep moving forward, she was excited to embark on the journey. She ended up ahead of schedule and left her job within nine months. Because she had prepared for this day, she was not nervous or scared about her future. Her business thrived and she was busier than she ever expected. She never imagined in her wildest dreams that she would be living this life. Her job was her passion and it did not even feel like work.

SIMPLIFIED HELP

"There is no way I can leave my job, I would be broke"

Remember what I said about being smart first, not jumping off the edge without a net. If leaving your current job is not a possibility right now, it does not mean you have to ignore your passions. Getting involved with an organization on a volunteer basis is a good start. By volunteering on a part-time basis you are meeting people and familiarizing yourself with the business. You are gaining skills and enjoying your time as well. You never know who you will meet or what opportunities will present themselves when you least expect it. You will also learn fairly quickly whether this job is something you would be interested in pursuing down the road. You may realize that you enjoy the work on the side, but it would not be a good fit as a professional endeavor. Do not give up hope that you will be able to pursue what you love. Just go at your own pace and create a path that fits your lifestyle now.

"I have no idea what I would love to do"

When long amounts of time pass during which you are not focusing on your natural abilities, you slowly forget what they are. That is exactly why it is imperative that you take some time to review your past. Start as a child if you have to. What did you do as a child that brought you joy? Did you love the theater and entertaining? Were you always fixing things around the house? Did your friends always come to you for advice? Your life is a blueprint if you can look deeply enough to see what it reveals. Start jotting down ideas and memories as they come to you. If you honestly cannot remember much from your past you will need to start fresh. Sign up for activities that spark your interest now. Get involved with people who have similar interests. Just get out there and see where the universe leads you. You may be pleasantly surprised.

SIMPLIFIED AFFIRMATIONS:

"I love my job and look forward to it every day"

"I am tapping into my natural strengths and passions"

"My work is an opportunity to experience joy"

"I trust that I will always be guided in the direction I need to go"

We spend a majority of our lives working, so you might as well do something you genuinely enjoy. I have been extremely blessed in my life. I have always pursued careers that utilize my strengths. I could never stay in something that made me miserable. The real estate business with my husband was exciting for a very short period of time, but then the emotional strain that I took on from all of our clients took its toll. I would stay up all night worrying whether or not their contract was going to be accepted. I was probably more anxious than the clients. I realized that I was far too invested in the outcome to be neutral and productive. I am grateful every day that I had the strength to realize this early on and do something about it.

I have a good friend who enjoyed the work she did, but she was extremely stressed and tense all the time. She was working very long hours and she missed her children. As a hands-on-mother this tug of war back and forth was driving her crazy. She felt guilty that she was not focused enough at work. She felt more guilt that she was missing out on experiences with her kids. To her this was a no-win situation. She did not want to quit work, for she genuinely enjoyed what she did. But she could not continue her schedule the way it was. She decided to talk with her boss and come up with a solution. They came up with an idea that solved many of the issues. She worked two long days and took the other three days to herself. She was working similar hours, but it allowed her more time to be with her family and friends on her days off. Instead of spreading work throughout the entire week, she now had designated hours. She was happy to create a compromise that worked for everyone. She had more time to nurture herself and take some down time. Her family was happier that she was home more and this alleviated some of the guilt.

Sometimes there is no one solution to every problem. I would love for you to find an answer that works for you. If you are unhappy at work, either seek new employment or get engaged in activities that bring you joy. There is always middle ground to explore. If you are unsure how to get started with pursuing a new career, there are many people who can be of assistance. You can work with a career counselor, a headhunter, a life coach or an executive coach. Any of these professionals will give you the tools and support to make the transition. Just remember to stick to your values and your natural strengths. There are some areas where you should not compromise. Good luck and congratulations on making it through to this chapter of the book!

Week 26

Zzz, take a deep breath and enjoy the new you!

Congratulations on reading this book in its entirety and making positive and lasting life changes. Each chapter is an opportunity for you to grow and evolve into the person you want to become. I want each and every one of you to know that no matter what expectation you put on yourself when you first started this book, you should be proud of what you *did* accomplish. This book should continue to act as your guide when life becomes challenging. Take some time and reflect on what you learned throughout this process. *What sticks out that had the biggest impact on you? Were there certain tools and exercises that you will continue to use in the future?* Fill in the blanks and see for yourself how you have evolved over the weeks.

I was able to simplify my life by _____

_____

Being in the moment means _____

_____

I am now more grateful for _____

_____

I will no longer allow fear to control _____

_____

By doing the following, I am able to get my needs met.

_____

_____

_____

_____

_____

_____

_____

I have come to realize that success to me looks like _____

_____

_____

The biggest change I have made in my life is _____

_____

_____

_____

I acknowledge myself for _____

_____

_____

_____

It is crucial to acknowledge everything you have accomplished. This is a critical step in building your self-worth and "confidence muscle." By recognizing everything you did, you are telling yourself that you can continue to rely on yourself to conquer fears and break through the unknown. If there were specific chapters that were a bit more difficult for you, you can always go back and spend more time working through them. I am committed to helping you improve your life, so I would like you to write down some personal goals that you would like to achieve by next year. You have a wonderful start to this process, and now I am pushing you a bit further. I want you to acknowledge everything you have achieved up to this point and then set the bar higher for the coming year. If you began to simplify your life, how can you continue this trend into the next year? If you created a life list, what can you do this year to cross off some of the items? I have given you an outline that you can duplicate onto another piece of paper. Making sure every goal is very specific, write each one down using the following outline:

Current date _____

Goal (I want to climb a fourteener) Be very specific here.

_____
_____
_____
_____
_____
_____
_____

Action steps (I will train twice a month with an endurance trainer and hike one time per month)

_____
_____
_____
_____
_____
_____
_____
_____
_____

When goal will be achieved (I will climb a fourteener by June 2009)

_____
_____
_____
_____

Is this an achievable goal? (Losing 20 pounds in one week is not realistic)

_____

_____

_____

Your goals need to be specific, measurable, realistic, and with a timeline attached. You have already proven to yourself that you can achieve anything you set your mind to, so keep up the good work. As I mentioned at the beginning of the book, I am not a believer in quick-fix remedies. I want you to make long-term lifestyle changes. Everything comes down to consistency, commitment, and a positive attitude. **Life Simplified** is meant to show you that you can make changes in your life without feeling overwhelmed or out of your league. Even if you take baby steps in the right direction, you are doing something you were not doing before. And in my mind that is progress.

Because this book was written in honor of my mother, I would like to share the most memorable life lessons that I learned from her. I embrace each one of them in my own life. Hopefully you can use these lessons as a guide in your own life.

* Follow your intuition as a way to steer you in the right direction

* Remember it is always ok to ask for help

* Each and every one of us has strength to carry us through the difficult times

* No matter how busy your life is, don't lose touch with the little moments that make up your life

* Lighten up and do not take life so seriously

* Always cultivate and nurture your friendships

* Find a balance in your life that feels right to you- there will always be a struggle, so just do your best

* Don't forget to take time for yourself

*Always learn and be open to evolving and growing as a person

I would like to thank each and every one of you for participating in this journey with me. I wish for you all a lifetime of happiness, freedom, fun and peace of mind. Life is such a blessing, so make sure you cherish it and nurture it. Continue your own journey of self discovery and remember that you can only do your best with the tools you are given. If you are unsure how to proceed, do not hesitate to ask for help. You can continue to check my website at www.newlifefocus.com for articles and support. Create your own Life Simplified support group and be proactive in creating your absolute best life. Keep up the great work and I look forward to hearing about the adventures that await you! Remember to always ***keep life simple***.

About Leslie Gail

Leslie Gail is a seasoned life coach with a wealth of experience, and has helped countless people transform their lives in positive ways. She has built her practice on the values of trust, passion and connection. Leslie received a Bachelor of Arts degree in Psychology prior to completing her life coaching certification. Leslie currently appears regularly on both radio and television. She appeared regularly on *KOSI-FM radio* in Denver as their lifestyle expert. Leslie also offered weekly 'tips' on *KMGH The Denver Channel*, as their official life coach. Leslie has published several articles in *Denver Woman magazine* and is a co-author of the book, *101 Great Ways to Improve your Life, Volume 3*. Leslie currently appears on *FOX31 Good Day Colorado*, offering simple and practical advice to their viewers. Leslie's passion is apparent in all that she does. She is able to connect with people at whatever crossroads they face. Leslie is an enthusiastic speaker who uses life experiences to connect with her audience. She currently resides in Colorado with her husband and two children.

To sign up for Leslie's free online newsletter, go to:
www.newlifefocus.com

E-mail Leslie directly at:
leslie@newlifefocus.com

If you would be interested in speaking with Leslie Gail regarding coaching services or speaking engagements, please contact:
1-866-779-0731

11140181R0011

Made in the USA
Lexington, KY
21 September 2011